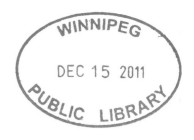
THE COMPLETE GUIDE TO
PHYSICAL ACTIVITY AND MENTAL HEALTH

Debbie Lawrence and Sarah Bolitho

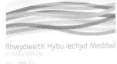

Rhwydwaith Hybu Iechyd Meddwl
CYMRU GYFAN
ALL WALES
Mental Health Promotion Network

Physical Activity and
Nutrition Networks Wales
Rhwydweithiau **Gweithgaredd**
Corfforol a Maeth Cymru

BTCV

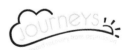

journeys

Note

Whilst every effort has been made to ensure that the content of this book is as technically accurate and as sound as possible, neither the author nor the publishers can accept responsibility for any injury or loss sustained as a result of the use of this material.

Published by A&C Black Publishers Ltd an imprint of
Bloomsbury Publishing Plc
49–51 Bedford Square
London
WC1B 3DP

First edition 2011

ISBN 978 1408 14021 5

Acknowledgements
Cover photograph © Shutterstock
Inside photographs © Shutterstock
Illustrations by David Gardner
Designed by James Watson
Commissioned by Charlotte Croft

This book is produced using paper that is made from wood grown in managed, sustainable forests. It is natural, renewable and recyclable. The logging and manufacturing processes conform to the environmental regulations of the country of origin.

Typeset in 10.75pt on 14pt Adobe Caslon by Saxon Graphics Ltd, Derby

Printed in Great Britain by Martins the Printers

// CONTENTS

FOREWORD

As a physiotherapist working in the Mental Health sector for more than 10 years I have seen the increasing importance of exercise for these patients in counteracting the poor lifestyle, higher morbidity rates from cardio-respiratory problems and diabetes and other side effects from medication that affects weight management and physical abilities. Stigma, prejudice and a lack of understanding impacts upon the ability of patients (or service users) to access services that may help them and they often require additional support to make the necessary changes.

Within health there are limited opportunities to participate in exercise and can be compromised due to the acuity of their illness. There is now an increasing focus on the recovery model and supporting service users in the community, and it is important that all exercise providers are able to provide suitable support to help patients to achieve their general health goals as part of their recovery and a healthy lifestyle. It will be essential to work collaboratively with healthcare providers that have an overlapping role with other providers to make the best use of all appropriate resources. This will include joint training of dedicated staff and identifying the smooth transfer of patients from hospital care to community focused care, dovetailing resources to ensure optimal recovery for the individual.

In the Mental Health sector, the transition between specialist exercise services for service users in secondary care provides an initial safe and supportive environment to help them get into a routine of exercising with a tailored approach, which in turn builds confidence and provides motivation. The advanced training of Level 4 practitioners gives me more confidence that the greater percentage of people with mental health problems that do not necessarily come into secondary care are supported by staff who understand in more depth how mental health affects an individual and their life. It will help reduce stigma and prejudice and aid social inclusion. It will also ensure that the principles of recovery and empowerment are incorporated into the engagement of people using exercise to regain their health and well-being.

Liz John
Head of Physiotherapy in Mental Health, Cardiff & Vale University Health Board
Member of the Chartered Society of Physiotherapy
2011

ACKNOWLEDGEMENTS

DEBBIE LAWRENCE

I give thanks to:

- My partner Joe for his patience, while I spent hours at the computer researching and writing this book.
- All the people (friends, family, clients) who have shared their own mental health and ill-health experiences and stories with me.
- My co-writer, Sarah, for working with me to produce this book.
- Fitness Wales for supporting the delivery of the Level 4 training programme, which this book supports.

'This book has been in the making for a long time, I hope it has arrived at a time when it can be most impactful and can make a difference to the way in which mental health is promoted and supported.'

SARAH BOLITHO

Thank you to:

- My family, especially my sister Anne who has been a strong support to me and my mother, who always looks out for the underdog.
- All the individuals and groups with mental health 'differences' that I have worked with over the last 20 years who have shown me that mental health problems are 'normal' conditions and something we need to accept not reject.
- My co-writer Debbie for making me do this!

'Having worked with individuals of all ages, backgrounds, abilities and disabilities with mental health conditions over the last 20 years, I hope that this book helps to both inform and encourage other instructors not only to work in this field, but also to learn more about their own mental health!'

INTRODUCTION

Over 300 people in every 1,000 experience mental health problems every year in Britain and of these 230 will visit a GP. From there, 102 people will be diagnosed as having a mental health problem and 24 will then be referred to a specialist psychiatric service with 6 becoming inpatients in psychiatric hospitals.

The aim of this book is to provide exercise professionals with the underpinning knowledge required to *design, agree, deliver and adapt physical activity and exercise programmes for persons with mental health conditions*.

The content is mapped to the National Occupational Standards at Level 4 (developed by SkillsActive 2010) and is designed to support the learning of exercise professionals who are working towards Level 4 qualification in Physical Activity for Persons with Mental Health Conditions.

The book does not provide explanations and descriptions of exercises or exercise programmes,

as these are detailed in other books from the Complete Guide and Fitness Professional series published by A & C Black. It is expected that instructors working towards any of the level 4 qualifications would hold qualifications in a range of level 2 and 3 exercise disciplines, to enable them to work in a variety of ways to support this client group becoming more active. Rather, this book will provide an overview of a range of mental health conditions and will discuss considerations for working with persons with these conditions. It will build on models of motivation and behavioural change and communication skills and explore ways of working with clients, including roles, responsibilities and boundaries, initial assessment and information gathering and planning and delivery considerations.

Debbie Lawrence
Sarah Bolitho
2011

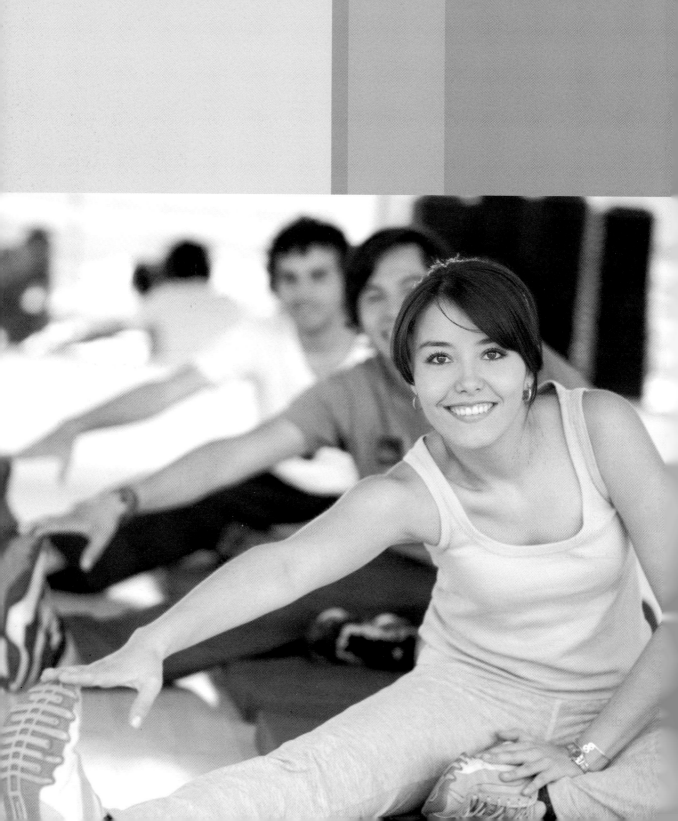

PART ONE

MENTAL HEALTH AND PHYSICAL ACTIVITY

Mental health is an aspect of our total health that is often taken for granted. We share our happy days and good moods and we celebrate our successes and joys. However it is a different story when we are feeling sad, grumpy or in emotional pain. Somehow these equally valid and important emotions are considered wrong, unpleasant and shameful. People are keen to share their happiness but all too often the less 'happy' emotions become internalised and locked away, unwanted and untreated.

This part aims to explore the concept of mental health and mental ill-health and to examine some of the theories surrounding mental health conditions. Also discussed are the more frequently encountered conditions, possible causes and available treatments, including activity.

The benefits of activity for mental health and the recommendations for participation are discussed and also examined are the barriers that exist, both internally and externally, that hinder the adoption of and adherence to physical activity.

It is hoped that this section will inspire you to consider your own mental health and to investigate your feelings about mental illness. As fitness professionals we have a role to play not only in promoting activity among individuals with mental health problems but also in developing awareness and understanding in others.

'During depression the world disappears. Language itself. One has nothing to say. Nothing. No small talk, no anecdotes. Nothing can be risked on the board of talk. Because the inner voice is so urgent in its own discourse: How shall I live? How shall I manage the future? Why should I go on?'
   – Kate Millett (1991) *The Loony Bin Trip*, Virago Press Ltd, UK

'Mental illness is nothing to be ashamed of, but stigma and bias shame us all.'
   – Bill Clinton

1

WHAT IS // MENTAL HEALTH? 1

This chapter introduces the concepts of mental health and mental illness. It outlines some definitions of mental health from varied and respected sources and introduces some of the factors that will affect our perception of what is considered normal and what is considered abnormal. With regard to mental health, this would include the beliefs, thoughts, attitudes, feelings/emotions, sensations and behaviours that are deemed as normal within our environment. These attitudes and beliefs will affect how we treat others with mental health conditions, also the regard in which we hold, and the value we place on, our own mental health.

This chapter also introduces some of the psychological models used to diagnose and treat mental health conditions. It outlines the criteria used by the medical classification system (DSM) and identifies some criticisms of this approach, setting the scene for a more integrative approach to working with clients with mental health conditions.

Ultimately, chapter 1 serves as an introduction to some of the themes and issues that will be revisited throughout the rest of the book.

OBJECTIVES

By the end of this chapter, you should be able to:

*   recognise some of the factors that contribute to the perception of what is normal/abnormal (thoughts, beliefs, attitudes, emotions, behaviours etc.) mental health;
*   recognise the psychological models and medical classification system used to define, diagnose and treat mental health conditions; and
*   recognise the integrative model as a holistic method.

DEFINING MENTAL HEALTH AND MENTAL ILLNESS

The terms 'mental health' and 'mental illness' probably conjure up a variety of images and hold different meanings for different people. If asked to answer the questions 'what is mental health?' and 'what is mental illness?' we may struggle to find clear definitions. Although our minds may be drawn to media and movie images depicting acts of behaviour that we may define as normal or abnormal in our world, *Webster's New World Dictionary* (4th edn., 1998) offers the following definitions:

- Mental: 'Pertaining to the mind. Effected by or due to the mind'
- Health: 'Soundness of any living organism. General condition of the body or mind, as to vigour and soundness'
- Illness: 'The state of being out of health. An ailment, sickness. Badness; evil'

These definitions provide a starting point, but in no way capture the wholeness of mental health, which is the more modern concept. Arguably, they may capture the essence of some of the generalised beliefs that exist with regard to mental illness – that it is abnormal, bad, evil, a taboo of society. Indeed, mental illness is a concept that has been recognised for centuries and throughout all civilisations and has been attributed to numerous causes, including witchcraft and possession by demonic spirits.

A number of organisations have offered definitions of mental health. The Health Education Authority (1997:5) describes being mentally healthy as having: '… the emotional and spiritual resilience which enables us to enjoy life and survive pain, disappointment and sadness. It is a positive sense of well-being and an underlying belief in our own and others' dignity and worth'

The Mental Health Foundation defines mental health as: 'A state of well-being in which the individual realises his or her own abilities, can cope with the normal stresses of life, can work productively and fruitfully, and is able to make a contribution to his or her community.' (See www.mentalhealth.org.uk for more information.)

In keeping with these definitions, Jackson and Hill, eds (2006:5) emphasise good mental health as the ability to:

Good mental health (Jackson and Hill, eds, 2006:5)

- Start, keep and if necessary, end relationships
- Work or attend college/school
- Look after oneself and others
- Sleep
- Laugh and cry
- Eat
- Avoid problems with substances
- Deal with what others think about you
- Accept failure and deal with success
- Function sexually, if wished
- Learn
- Deal with loss
- Express good feelings
- Manage negative feelings

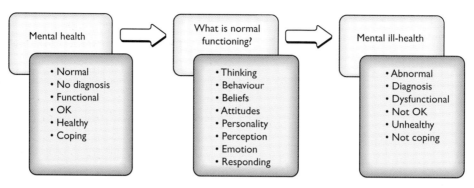

Figure 1.1 Single continuum model of mental health

NORMAL OR ABNORMAL MENTAL WELL-BEING

The continuum model indicates that mental health and mental ill-health are single dimensional entities. Using this model, classification of an individual's mental well-being would probably teeter somewhere between the polar extremes of what psychiatric experts might refer to as being *functional* (healthy) and *dysfunctional* (not healthy). This relates to thinking, perception, responding, behaviour, personality, intellect and emotion; those aspects of functioning that are not specific to a bodily or physiological system, such as gastro-intestinal and respiratory functioning (Daines et al., 1997) (see Figure 1.1).

However, there is no clear, single boundary that creates a defining point between what is considered positive mental health and what is considered mental ill-health or mental illness.

A psychiatrist generally uses the term 'mental illness' when there are a clear range of signs and symptoms (referred to as a 'syndrome') present and where there is a distinct deterioration in the person's functioning (Daines et al., 1997). Some of the factors that contribute to the controversy of

defining where the 'cut-off point' is are introduced later in this chapter (see page 16), along with references to the classification systems currently used to assess mental health.

An alternative model to the single continuum model is the dual continuum model. This model reflects a shift in awareness in that health is not merely the absence of disease or illness; it is more than that. This model accepts that a 'mentally healthy person can become depressed under certain circumstances; just as a physically healthy person can acquire an injury or infection' (Jackson and Hill, 2006:3). It also indicates that a person with a diagnosis of a mental health condition can function quite *normally*, provided they receive appropriate care and support, as would a person with a physical health condition. From this perspective, mental health is therefore a *dynamic state* that can change in response to circumstances within our world and includes our subjective personal experiencing and the impact of our environment (community) on our experience. It is not something that can be exclusively classified by only external measures alone (diagnosis) (see Figure 1.2).

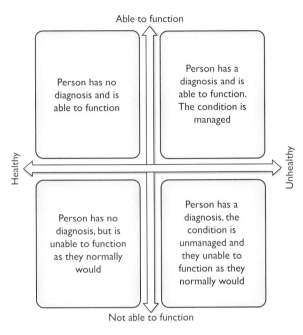

Figure 1.2 Dual continuum of mental health

Able to function

Person has no diagnosis and is able to function

Person has a diagnosis and is able to function. The condition is managed

Healthy

Unhealthy

Person has no diagnosis, but is unable to function as they normally would

Person has a diagnosis, the condition is unmanaged and they unable to function as they normally would

Not able to function

PREVALENCE OF MENTAL HEALTH CONDITIONS

It may be a common belief that mental health conditions affect only a few people, making it their own problem, rather than a broader issue. Unfortunately this is not the case. In fact, the World Health Organisation (WHO) forecasts that depression will be second only to coronary heart disease as the leading contributor to the global burden of disease by the year 2020 (MHF, 2007:10).

To offer some perspective of the prevalence of mental health conditions, the Mental Health Foundation (2007/2010) reported the following statistics:

- 1 in 4 British adults experience at least one diagnosable mental health problem in a year.
- Mixed anxiety and depression is the most common condition in Britain, affecting approximately 9 per cent of people.
- Between 8 and 12 per cent of the population experience depression in any year.
- Women are twice as likely to experience anxiety as men are.
- An estimated 121 million worldwide will experience a depressive episode in a year.
- 60 per cent of people with phobias or obsessive-compulsive disorder (OCD) are female.
- Phobias affect 22 in 1,000 women and 13 in 1,000 men.
- 2–3 per cent of people will experience obsessive-compulsive disorder during their lifetime.
- Approximately 1 in 200 adults experience probable psychotic disorder in the course of a year, with the average age of onset of psychotic symptoms being 22.
- Schizophrenia is the most common of the psychotic disorders, affecting between 1.1 per cent and 2.4 per cent of people at any single time.
- 25 per cent of people with schizophrenia will make a full recovery, while 10–15 per cent will experience severe long-term effects.
- 1.7 per cent of adults worldwide have an alcohol-use disorder.
- In the year 2000, a quarter of adults in the UK were assessed as consuming alcohol at 'hazardous' levels.
- 80 per cent of persons dependent on alcohol, 75 per cent of people dependent on cannabis and 69 per cent of those dependent on other illegal drugs are male.
- 1 in 4 unemployed people has a common mental health problem.

- 1 in 10 children between the ages of 1 and 15 has a mental health disorder.
- It is estimated that approximately 450 million people worldwide have a mental health problem (WHO, 2001).
- Women are more likely to have been treated for a mental health problem than men.
- Depression is more common in women than in men.
- Dementia affects 5 per cent of people over the age of 65 and 20 per cent of those over 80.
- Mental health problems are thought to be higher in minority ethnic groups than in the white population, but these groups are less likely to have their mental health problems detected by a GP.
- Rates of mental health problems among children increase as they reach adolescence.
- Depression affects 1 in 5 older people living in the community and 2 in 5 living in care homes.
- In 2004 more than 5,500 people in the UK died by suicide.
- British men are three times as likely as British women to die by suicide.
- Suicide remains the most common cause of death in men under the age of 35.
- The suicide rate in prisons is almost 15 times higher than in the general population.
- The UK has one of the highest rates of self-harm in Europe, at 400 per 100,000 population.
- More than 70 per cent of the prison population has two or more mental health disorders. Male prisoners are 14 times more likely to have two or more disorders than men in general, and female prisoners 35 times more likely than women in general.
- Anorexia nervosa will be experienced by 1 per cent and 0.2 per cent of men in any year.
- Bulimia affects between 0.5 per cent and 1 per cent of women.

Statistics on Mental Health are from the MHF website 2010 (www.mentalhealth.org.uk/information/mental-health-overview/statistics/) and MHF Fundamental Facts (2007).

With these statistics in mind, mental health conditions may be more common and more 'normal' than we may initially think they are.

PERCEPTIONS OF MENTAL ILLNESS

Whether we know it or not, it is highly likely we will all know someone who has experienced or is experiencing a mental health condition – with an estimated 1 in 4 adults experiencing a condition in any year, we arguably would not need to look outside our family or workplace.

Unfortunately, mental health conditions are still taboo for many people. While most people would comfortably visit a personal trainer to help them get their body fit, speak with a GP about a medical condition, or ask for help from a dietician to improve their eating habits and diet, very few would have the same willingness and enthusiasm for visiting a counsellor or psychotherapist to help with their mind and emotions. Yet mental and emotional fitness are important aspects of our overall health, well-being and total fitness.

There is still much stigma attached to mental health and mental illness. It seems that physical ill-health or illness is OK whereas mental ill-health or illness is *not* OK. Modern campaigns, such as time4change (a campaign in England) supported by Mind, the Mental Health Foundation and other organisations, is attempting to change this general attitude.

STEREO-TYPING/LABELLING

Classifying and diagnosing a person as having a specific mental condition is intended as a guide and starting point to assisting with the planning of their treatment. However, there appears to be a general lack of awareness, fear, discomfort and ignorance around the experience of persons with mental and emotional distress. When a person is classified or diagnosed as having a mental illness it can often lead to others adopting stereotypical views towards that person(s), which can cause them to feel separated and excluded (see Figure 1.3).

The Mental Health Foundation (2005) reports that 70 per cent of persons with mental health conditions have experienced discrimination (56 per cent have experienced discrimination from family and 52 per cent from friends, 44 per cent from their GP and 32 per cent from a healthcare professional). It is therefore perhaps not unsurprising that 42 per cent choose not to tell friends or family about their condition, which means they are lacking crucial support at a time when they most need it (see Figure 1.4).

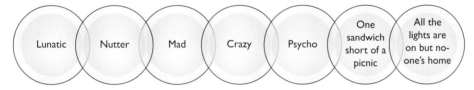

Figure 1.3 Negative labelling

'Mental health problems are for weak people'
Err ... what about Winston Churchill, Abraham Lincoln, Stephen Fry, Ruby Wax, Alistair Campbell...

'You won't get anywhere in life with a mental health problem'
Tell that to the people mentioned above and to Patsy Palmer, Billy Joel, Woody Allen, Charles Dickens, John Lennon...

'I don't know anyone with mental health problem'
One in four people in the UK will experience a mental health problem so it is likely that you actually know several people who have, or have had, a mental health problem

'Mental ill people are violent'
In fact violent acts are rarely committed by people with mental health problems, they are far more likely to hurt themselves than others or be attacked by members of the public because of their condition

'Once you have a mental health problem you can't get rid of it'
Not true, with appropriate treatment it is possible to overcome many mental health problems and return to a 'normal life'

Figure 1.4 Common misconceptions about mental health disorders

Figure 1.4 tackles some of the common misconceptions about mental health disorders.

Unfortunately, it is still a sad fact that disclosing a mental health disorder – even from the distant past – can result in a job offer suddenly being withdrawn or downgraded, or a current employee being suddenly made redundant. The MHF (2005) indicates that 39 per cent of adults with mental health conditions were unemployed compared with the general unemployment figure of 7.7 per cent. This is another reason that many people hide mental health problems when applying for work, but this in itself can lead to further problems if they are under stress or have a relapse, as they may not want to approach the organisation for help or support.

Indeed, mental health issues, such as depression and stress, are now the largest condition group where absenteeism and incapacity benefit are concerned. This is despite the Health and Safety Executive (HSE) guidelines on stress management in the workplace and the requirements of the Equalities Act 2010, which includes long-term mental illness as a category of disability.

MENTAL ILLNESS, THE MEDIA AND CRIME

The media has frequently been criticised for the way in which it reports and portrays persons with mental health conditions, and especially its tendency to link mental illness with criminal violence. It has been suggested that this compounds some of the discrimination and prejudice that people with mental health conditions face.

In fact, there is evidence to suggest that this is not an accurate representation. The National Institute of Mental Health (NIMH, 2010) indicates that persons with schizophrenia are not prone to violence; with the exception being those persons who have a criminal record before becoming ill or those with substance and alcohol abuse problems. They add that people with schizophrenia are not usually violent, preferring to be left alone, and that most violent crimes are committed by persons who do not have schizophrenia. NIMH (2010) suggests that substance abuse may raise the rate of violence, but this applies to people both with and without schizophrenia.

In reality, most violent offences are committed by individuals who do not have a mental health disorder. Of the 757 homicides in the UK in 2005, fewer than 10 per cent were committed by a person with a mental illness. In contrast, MHF (2005) reported that 1 in 7 persons with mental health conditions had been physically attacked and 50 per cent had been abused or harassed. In reality, most people with a severe mental health problem are more likely to harm themselves than another person. Unfortunately, the perception that someone with a mental health condition is 'dangerous' persists and serves only to increase stigma, prejudice and discrimination.

Further perceptions held by the general public towards persons with one of the more common mental health problems were reported in a survey by the Royal College of Psychiatrists. It was found that:

- 74 per cent rated drug addicts as dangerous while 71 per cent thought schizophrenics were a threat and 65 per cent believed alcoholics to be a danger.
- 49 per cent of people thought those with severe depression should 'pull themselves together'.

- 47 per cent thought drug addicts were to blame for their illness while 33 per cent thought the same of alcoholics and 39 per cent thought the same for people with eating disorders.
- 81 per cent of people thought alcoholics were unpredictable, compared with 78 per cent for drug addicts and 77 per cent for schizophrenics, and around 56 per cent of people with severe depression and 50 per cent of those suffering panic attacks were described as unpredictable.
- A majority believed the condition of people with dementia will not improve with treatment; 16 per cent believed depression could not be treated, compared with 15 per cent for schizophrenia, 14 per cent for panic attacks, 12 per cent for drug addiction, 11 per cent for alcoholism and 10 per cent for eating disorders.
- Many people still think it is difficult to communicate with people with mental illness.

Stereotyping, labelling and prejudice are not helpful as they can contribute towards impeding a person's recovery. They can also prevent people from seeking the help they need when experiencing mental and emotional distress. Interestingly, stereotyping in itself can also be viewed as 'pathological' (Gross and McIlveen, 1998:456). Indeed, many of the stereotypes portrayed are often 'contradicted by ordinary peoples' experiences of mental health problems affecting themselves, their family members, friends or work colleagues,' according to the MHF (Mental illness factsheet, 2000).

FACTORS INFLUENCING PERCEPTION

The beliefs and attitudes we hold in relation to 'being okay' are influenced by a number of factors, some of which are outlined in Figure 1.5.

Social and cultural factors

The way a person thinks and feels about and behaves towards issues of mental health and mental illness, and the way they respond to specific life events and circumstances, is highly influenced by the cultural and social group to which they belong and the way they react to the experience of life and living.

Social and cultural 'norms' influence many things including how we dress (the burkha, the bikini or body piercings), how we speak (voice tone and volume, the words we use, whether it be

Case study

'My uncle Bob had schizophrenia. On reflection, I always found his behaviour really odd. His eyes usually had a glazed look (probably the medications) and he was for the most part 'expressionless', which made it harder for me to understand him. He chain-smoked, rarely went out, usually drank too much at Christmas and was dependent on family for care for all of his life. He recently died, in his late seventies, after spending the last few years of his life undergoing kidney dialysis.

He was different, but he was never violent. In fact, my Mum reported a number of occasions when his home was robbed and he was conned out of money (to clean windows or do gardening) by tricksters. These stories get less if any mileage in the media!'

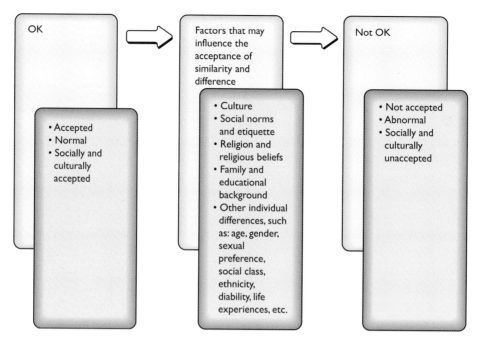

Figure 1.5 Factors influencing the perception of normal

slang or swearing), how we behave (diet, exercise, the work we choose, our attitude to work, education, socialisation), sexual preference (heterosexual, homosexual, bi-sexual, transgender, transsexual etc.), religious beliefs or spiritual beliefs. Furthermore, what is considered 'normal' (and accepted) by one culture, social group or system (including families and organisations) can often be seen as 'abnormal' (and unaccepted) by another culture and/or social group.

Social and cultural 'norms' also have a tendency to 'shift' and change over time. For example, in the Middle Ages it was normal to believe that a person with a birthmark or mole was a witch and that they had made a pact with the devil. The person's 'purity' was assessed by ducking them in water using a ducking stool, a common ritual of the day. It was thought that those who sank were pure and

those who kept their head above the water (floated) were impure. The outcome of this ritual was that those deemed pure actually drowned (they sank) and those deemed impure were rescued from the ducking, only to be burned at the stake (Gross & McIlveen, 1998:568).

The point is that when we are referring to concepts such as normal and abnormal, we need to maintain an open mind. This is particularly important in a multi-cultural society, where similarities and differences between different cultural groups need to be explored and embraced as a difference, rather than an abnormality. Those interested in reading further into the area of difference in relation to various cultural groups are referred to the ideas and viewpoints expressed by Fernando (1988), Gross and McIlveen (1998:562-613), Lago & Thompson (2003), Mindell (1995) and Rack (1982) which are listed in the references (see page 192).

DIAGNOSING MENTAL ILLNESS

Within the field of human psychology and behaviour, there are a number of models which contribute ideas and theories towards what constitutes 'mental ill-health'. These include the following: biological/medical, genetic, psycho-dynamic, behavioural, cognitive, humanistic, social, systemic, intuitive and existential. Each of the major models promotes a different set of theories of how mental, emotional and behavioural disturbances can occur and how they should be treated to promote recovery. Each model probably offers an aspect of the *truth* regarding the origin for mental health problems and their best treatment. Therefore an integrated/eclectic approach, where all models are considered, is arguably more holistic (see Figure 1.6).

THE MEDICAL MODEL

The most influential model for classifying mental health conditions has been the medical model, which identifies collections of signs and symptoms (a syndrome) that lead to diagnosis of specific mental conditions against the specific classificatory systems. Early contributors included Hippocrates, Asclepiades and Pinel. However, it was a later contributor, Kraepelin (1913), who collated and elaborated on the information provided by earlier systems to provide a more comprehensive system for diagnosing mental health. Kraepelin elaborated on the earlier systems by observing hospitalised patients and their records and from this proposed 18 distinct types of mental disorder, each with a

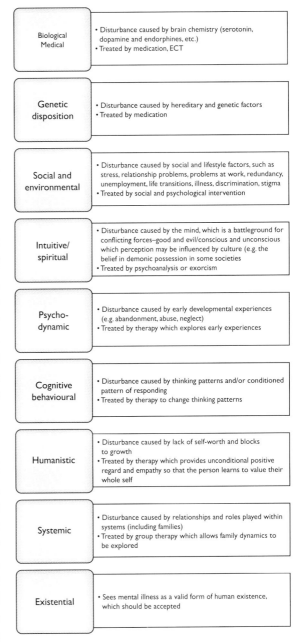

Figure 1.6 Psychological models

characteristic set of symptoms (a syndrome) (Gross and Mcilveen 1998: 575). The WHO was created in 1948 and the ICD and DSM were published shortly after this. The 1983 Mental Health Act embodies Kraepelins system and identifies three categories of mental disturbance as: mental illness, personality disorder and mental impairment.

The medical model implies that mental health problems are primarily caused by biological and medical factors; hence treatment plans tend to rely heavily on medication. The two current medical classification and diagnostic systems (International Statistical Classification of Diseases and Related Health Problems 10th Revision (ICD-10) and the Diagnostic and Statistical Manual of Mental Disorders, 4th edition, text revision (DSM-IV-TR) have been developed from the work of Kraepelin.

An overview of the different categories of mental conditions that are classified on the ICD-10 and DSM-IV-TR are listed below.

The ICD-10 is an international standard diagnostic system of classification for a variety of health conditions and disorders and is produced by the WHO (see Figure 1.7, page 13).

The DSM-IV-TR is published by the American Psychiatric Association (1952) and characterises mental disorders. It states that 'there is no assumption that each category of mental disorder is a completely discrete entity with absolute boundaries dividing it from other mental disorders or from no mental disorder'. The DSM is clear that what is being classified is *a disorder that a person may have*, it is not the classification of a person (see Table 1.1).

The DSM is a multiaxial system that allows a comprehensive and systematic evaluation of the patient, involving an assessment on several axes. This can help not only with assessment but also with a treatment plan. There are five axes in the DSM on which disorder can be assessed:

Axis I: Clinical disorders and other conditions that may be a focus of clinical attention

Axis I is used to report the majority of mental health disorders, with the exception of personality disorders and mental retardation that are covered in Axis II.

Axis II: Personality disorders and mental retardation

Axis II covers personality disorders and mental retardation (learning disability).

Axis III: General medical conditions

This Axis relates to general medical conditions that may be relevant to an individual's mental health disorder. Medical conditions may link to mental health problems in a number of ways. There may be a clear link between the medical condition and the development or worsening of mental health symptoms, for example, depression with hypothyroidism or menopause, or there may be a reaction to a medical condition, for example, following a diagnosis of a life-threatening or serious condition such as cancer or HIV.

Axis IV: Psychosocial and environmental problems

Psychosocial or environmental problems may affect how a mental health condition is diagnosed, treated or managed and can have an impact on the prognosis. These factors include negative life events such as bereavement, or a lack of social or

Organic, including symptomatic, mental disorders

- Dementias, delirium, disorders due to brain disease, damage and dysfunction

Mental and behavioural disorders due to psychoactive substance use

- Disorders due to alcohol, cannabinoids, cocaine and hallucinogens

Schizophrenia, schizotypal and delusional disorders

- Schizophrenia, schizotypal and schizoaffective disorder, delusional disorder, psychotic disorder

Mood affective disorders

- Manic episode, bipolar affective disorder, depressive episode, recurrent depressive disorder, persistent mood (affective) disorder

Neurotic, stress-related and somotoform disorder

- Phobia anxiety disorders, obsessive compulsive disorder, post-traumatic stress disorder, adjustment disorder

Behavioural syndromes associated with physiological disturbances and physical factors

- Eating disorders, non-organic sleep disorders, non-organic sexual dysfunction, postnatal depression

Disorders of adult personality and behaviour

- Specific personality disorders, habit and impulse disorders, gender and identity disorders, disorders of sexual preference

Mental retardation

- Learning disability or intellectual disability

Disorders of psychological development

- Speech and language development disorders, scholastic development disorders (reading and writing), pervasive development disorders (autism)

Behavioural and emotional disorders, with onset usually in childhood

- Hyperkinetic disorders, conduct disorders, emotional disorders, tic disorders

Unspecified mental disorders

Figure 1.7 Overview ICD-10 classification system for mental disorders, chapter V(F), which specifically examines mental and behavioural disorders

Table 1.1	The main categories of disorder in the DSM-IV-TR classification system
DSM category	**Includes**
Disorders usually first diagnosed in infancy, childhood and adolescence	Attention deficit hyperactivity disorder (ADHD) (NB: Category excludes mental retardation)
Delirium, dementia, and amnestic and other cognitive disorders	Alzheimer's disease
Mental disorders due to a general medical condition	AIDS-related psychosis
Substance-related disorders	Alcohol misuse
Schizophrenia and other psychotic disorders	Schizophrenia
Mood disorders	Depression; bipolar disorder
Anxiety disorders	Generalised anxiety disorder; agoraphobia stress; panic disorder; specific phobia obsessive-compulsive disorder (OCD); social phobia; post-traumatic stress disorder (PTSD)
Somatoform disorders	Hysteria; body dysmorphic disorder; hypochondriasis
Factitious disorders	Munchausen syndrome
Dissociative disorders	Dissociative identity disorder; dissociative fugue
Sexual and gender identity disorders	Gender identity disorder; premature ejaculation; exhibitionism; voyeurism
Eating disorders	Anorexia nervosa; bulimia nervosa; binge-eating disorder
Sleep disorders	Insomnia; narcolepsy
Impulse-control disorders not elsewhere classified	Kleptomania; pyromania; trichotillimania
Adjustment disorders	Adjustment disorder
Personality disorders	Paranoid personality disorder; schizoid personality disorder; schizotypal personality disorder; antisocial personality disorder; borderline personality disorder; histrionic personality disorder; narcissistic personality disorder; avoidant personality disorder; dependent personality disorder; obsessive-compulsive personality disorder; personality disorder not otherwise specified
Other conditions that may be a focus of clinical attention	Psychological factor affecting medical condition medication-induced movement disorders; relational problems; problems relating to abuse or neglect; other additional conditions

familial support or of personal coping resources, including the following:

- Problems with primary support group
- Problems related to the social environment
- Educational problems
- Occupational problems
- Housing problems
- Economic problems
- Problems with access to health care services
- Problems related to interaction with the legal system or crime
- Other psychosocial and environmental problems

Axis V: Global assessment of functioning (GAF)

A clinician will use the GAF to assess an individual's level of functioning or ability to cope and use this information to plan treatment and management of the condition.

CRITICISMS, OBSERVATIONS AND COMPLAINTS OF DSM-IV (1994)

There have been a number of criticisms of the medical model over the years. Some of these include the following:

- It reduces human beings to one-dimensional sources of data; it does not encourage practitioners to treat the whole person.
- It perpetuates the social stigma attached to mental disorders.
- The symptom-based criteria sets of DSM-IV have led to an endless multiplication of mental conditions and disorders. The unwieldy size of DSM-IV is a common complaint of doctors in clinical practice – a volume that was only 119 pages long in its second edition (1968) has swelled to 886 pages in less than 30 years.

- The symptom-based approach has also made it easier to politicise the process of defining new disorders for inclusion or exclusion. The inclusion of post-traumatic stress disorder (PTSD) and the deletion of homosexuality as a disorder are often cited as examples of this concern for political correctness.
- The criteria sets do not allow for ordinary diversity among people. Some of the diagnostic categories of DSM-IV come close to defining various temperamental and personality differences as mental disorders.
- It does not distinguish adequately between poor adaptation to ordinary problems of living and true psychopathology. One by-product of this inadequacy is the suspiciously high rates of prevalence reported for some mental disorders. One observer remarked that ' … it is doubtful that 28 per cent or 29 per cent of the population would be judged [by managed care plans] to need mental health treatment in a year'.
- The 16 major diagnostic classes defined by DSM-IV hinder efforts to recognise disorders that run across classes. For example, PTSD has more in common with respect to aetiology and treatment with the dissociative disorders than it does with the anxiety disorders with which it is presently grouped. Another example is body dysmorphic disorder, which resembles the obsessive-compulsive disorders more than it does the somatoform disorders.
- It is deficient in acknowledging disorders of uncontrolled anger, hostility and aggression. Even though inappropriate expressions of anger and aggression lie at the roots of major social problems, only one DSM-IV disorder

(intermittent explosive disorder, within the category of impulse control disorders not elsewhere classified in the table above) is explicitly concerned with them. In contrast, entire classes of disorders are devoted to depression and anxiety.

• The emphasis of DSM-IV on biological psychiatry has contributed to the widespread popular notion that most problems of human life can be solved by 'taking pills'.

Source: www.minddisorders.com/Del-Fi/Diagnostic-and-Statistical-Manual-of-Mental-Disorders.html.

Persons interested in reading further criticisms are directed to Bentau, R (2010) *Doctoring the Mind: why psychiatric treatments fail.*

As the MHF (2010) suggests, most mental health problems result from a complex interaction of a range of biological, social and personal factors. People with mental health conditions are human beings and often share common feelings including guilt, shame, anxiety, fear and confusion about their condition and themselves. They may also share various potential risk factors and 'possible' causes, which include anxiety, poor parenting, genetic predisposition and substance misuse. Add the 'commonality' of concurrent physical ill-health (comorbidities) and arguably a more integrative way of working and the offer of a more holistic approach to treatment is the way forward (Jackson & Hill, 2006:8).

With this in mind, while diagnosis of a specific condition can guide the planning of medical treatment, other contributory factors, such as social support systems, impact of stressful life events etc. should also be considered for guiding treatment plans. As Daines et al. (1997:68) suggests, 'No single model can provide all the answers, so an experienced psychiatrist learns the value of eclecticism of working as part of a team' within both primary care (a GP, practice nurse, counsellor, exercise on referral professional) and secondary care (a psychologist, social worker).

TOWARDS AN INTEGRATIVE APPROACH – BEYOND THE MEDICAL MODEL

Most of the guidance provided by the National Institute for Health and Clinical Excellence (NICE) for the treatment of mental health conditions suggests a combination of possible interventions and treatments that may help the person to recover. All guidance is updated regularly and is supported by a specific evidence base and research. Some of the interventions listed for some mental health conditions include (depending on the condition and availability of intervention): hospitalisation, medication, diet and exercise (including exercise referral by GPs), therapeutic interventions and counselling, life skills training, a community care approach etc. Indeed, most people with mental health conditions respond best to holistic treatments, yet 'integrated care is hardly ever available in statutory services' (Jackson & Hill, 2006:8).

In support of an integrative approach to working with clients with mental health conditions, Jackson & Hill (2006:8) suggest that practitioners need to view the different medical models as 'complementary, rather than conflicting'. They suggest that the models can be understood by grouping them into the four dimensions shown in table 1.2 and that integrative treatment plans should take account of each of

Table 1.2	Dimensions of mental illness, adapted from Wilber (2000) in Jackson & Hill, eds (2006:9)	
	Subjective	**Objective**
Individual/self	'I'	'It'
	The individual	The health professionals
	Interior – as seen from the inside	Exterior – as seen from the outside
	Individual therapeutic models	Medical model
	(intervention, e.g. psychoanalysis)	(intervention, e.g. cognitive behavioural therapy (CBT), drugs)
Collective/self and others	'We'	'They'
	Family, community and society	Community and society
	Citizens	Exterior collective
	Interior collective	Policy makers
	Group therapeutic models	Health promotion
	(intervention, e.g. group therapy)	(intervention, e.g. anti-bullying strategies in schools)

these 'quadrants'. This should include the objective measures offered by the DSM-IV-TR and ICD-10 medical model, the subjective experiencing of the individual, including their experience in the community, and the perceptions/attitudes of others in their community towards them and towards mental health in general.

However, as Jackson & Hill (2006:9) suggest, 'an integrated future depends on non-medical practitioners being aware of the limits of their own influence' (the roles, responsibilities and boundaries of an exercise professional are explored in chapter 6). Persons specialising in psychiatry, psychology and medicine should acknowledge that their special knowledge, while vital, is only partial. A joint approach to working and the provision of holistic integrated care should involve collaboration between:

• medical and psychiatric professionals;

• non-medical professionals, who have complimentary specialist knowledge (e.g. exercise-on-referral professionals); and

• persons who have reflected on their own lived experience of mental health conditions (service users) or who have delivered practical help to others with mental health conditions (carers, relatives, friends) (Jackson & Hill, 2006:8).

TOWARDS THE RECOVERY MODEL APPROACH

Numerous legislation written over the last decade reports on: the health inequalities experienced by specific socio-economic groups; the impact of reduced physical activity on mental and medical health; and the additional burden of ill-health (physical and mental) on the National Health Service (NHS).

Physical activity is promoted as a medium for improving health in many of these government policies and initiatives and forms part of the recovery movement. This movement is a movement towards collaborative working and the provision of holistic integrated care involving medical professionals, service users and carers and other non-medical health practitioners (exercise professionals and counsellors) with the aim being to assist recovery. Some of the evidence and legislation that supports the use of physical activity and exercise as part of a treatment plan for mental illness within primary care is discussed in throughout this book .

SUMMARY POINTS

You should now be able to:

- List and explain some of the factors that will affect an individual's perception of what is considered to be normal, with regard to mental health.
- Describe the medical model of classification.
- Describe other models/theories that classify mental health.
- Summarise the integrative approach to working.

MENTAL HEALTH CONDITIONS

2

This chapter introduces and describes some of the main mental health conditions classified and introduces a range of treatment interventions.

The suggested exercise prescriptions (American College of Sports Medicine (ACSM) and Department of Health (DoH) etc.) should be considered, as always, with reference to the specific needs of the individual, including fitness levels, medication and comorbidities as these may have a significant impact on the exercise and/or activity intervention.

A further consideration is that any exercise professional should respect their boundary of competence and should only plan and deliver qualifications and services for which they are qualified and for which they are employed to conduct.

OBJECTIVES

By the end of this chapter you should be able to:

* recognise a range of classified mental health conditions;
* recognise the signs and symptoms of each condition;
* recognise the effects of each condition on physiological systems (neurological, muscular skeletal, cardiovasular (CV), respiratory, endocrine);
* recognise comorbidities that may exist with specific mental health conditions (obesity, high blood pressure, chronic obstructive pulmonary disease (COPD), other mental health conditions etc.);
* recognise factors which may contribute to the development of each condition;
* recognise a range of interventions and treatments for each condition;
* recognise the physiological effects of different medications used to treat specific mental health conditions; and
* review and discuss the ACSM and NICE/DoH exercise guidelines for specific conditions.

DEPRESSION AND MOOD DISORDERS

Depressive disorders are conditions that embrace a wide range of signs and symptoms that adversely affect the body (physical and behavioural), thinking (mental) and mood (emotional). Depressive disorders are not the same as a passing low mood, as they can cause more serious problems that impact upon daily living (how a person eats, sleeps, thinks and feels about themselves and the world and how they cope) and in severe instances they can lead to suicide.

Of all the psychological disorders, depression is the one most commonly seen by GPs. WHO ranks it as one of the leading causes of years lived with a disability worldwide and places it second only to ischemic heart disease in developed countries.

Depression

Depression is not a condition of the weak. There are a number of famous people who have experienced depresssion. To name but a few, these include Isaac Newton, Abraham Lincoln, Winston Churchill, Vincent van Gogh, Spike Milligan, Tony Hancock and Ernest Hemingway.

DEFINITION

Depression is defined as a pervasive lowering of mood with three core symptoms: low mood, anhedonia and decreased energy (see below).

SYMPTOMS

There are a number of clinical features of depression that fit broadly into three categories:

1   **Emotional:** Depression affects a person's mental state in a number of ways including low mood, feelings of excessive guilt, worthlessness or pointlessness, negative thought content and even delusions. There may be a diurnal variation in symptoms, with a lower mood in the morning than the evening. Further symptoms include suicide ideation or thoughts of death or thinking that the person would be better off dead. These cognitive effects can lead to perceptive selectivity – seeing only what suits the mood, usually negative, and perpetuating a cycle of negative thought.

2   **Anhedonic:** These symptoms involve the loss of enjoyment of previously enjoyable activities, usually accompanied by a loss of motivation and emotional reactions. Commonly, libido is significantly affected, which can cause additional problems in relationships if the presence of depression is not known.

3   **Physical:** Common physical symptoms or effects of depression include changes in sleep patterns and quality and increased or decreased appetite with associated weight gain or loss. Changes in motor activity may be present, with psychomotor retardation or agitation a common symptom. Psychomotor skills relate to those tasks that are performed so often that their execution is unconscious, such as walking, talking, riding a bike, tasks of self-care, etc. A slowing down (retardation) or agitation of psychomotor ability will result in everyday tasks becoming much more difficult due to slowing down or speeding up so they are ineffective, or possibly dangerous.

PREVALENCE

According to the MHF, 1 in 4 women and 1 in 10 men will experience an episode of depression serious enough to require treatment at some point in their life (Halliwell, 2005:13). The ratio of women to men experiencing depression is approximately 2:1 (Strock, 2000). This may be due to hormonal factors that affect women (menstruation, pregnancy, birth, etc.) and/or other responsibilities (caring for children and/or elderly relatives, work). Alternatively, Strock (2000) suggests that depression in men may be 'masked by alcohol and drugs' and that men are less likely to admit feeling depressed. She also suggests that depression in men tends to be displayed as irritability and anger and men often may be less inclined to ask for help.

It is estimated that over 20 per cent of individuals with major depression never seek help or are seen by their GP and that for 40 per cent of those with depression who do visit their GP, it is not recognised because they present with other physical illnesses or symptoms that may mask the psychological signs of the condition (Daines et al., 1997). It is also possible that people may lack the awareness of the warning signs (lack of self-awareness) or are reluctant to admit to feeling mentally unwell, perhaps hoping their GP will 'guess'.

Approximately 15 per cent of severely depressed adults commit suicide, with anti-depressant overdose implicated in up to 10 per cent of cases.

DIFFERENT TYPES OF DEPRESSION
Major clinical depression
A major depressive episode can occur only once but more frequently occurs more than once throughout a life span. People with major depression lose their zest for life and pleasure and lose the motivation to take care of themselves. Without treatment, the symptoms can last for months or years (Strock, 2000). It is estimated that within five years of suffering a major episode, a quarter of sufferers will attempt suicide.

Seasonal affective disorder (SAD)
SAD is a common form of depression and is linked to a lack of sunlight. It generally starts once the summer season has ended, and is present during autumn and winter, with symptoms easing in spring when daylight hours increase and sunshine starts to re-appear. People who work in offices sometimes use special lights over their PC screens that are designed to treat SAD. There is no definitive cause or trigger of SAD, however low serotonin levels or high melatonin levels and a disrupted body clock are all linked to the functioning of the hypothalamus, which is implicated in mood control. The onset of SAD may be linked to life events such as bereavement, illness or childbirth.

SAD is rare near the equator but common in the rest of the world. Estimated to affect twice as many women as men, onset is typically between 18 and 30 years. Treatment is usually with bright light therapy and talking therapies may also be helpful.

Postnatal depression
Postnatal depression (PND) occurs after childbirth and the combined factors of both hormonal changes and the responsibilities of taking care of a newborn child may be causal factors. Onset can be any time in the first two years after birth and it is estimated that 1 in 10 new mothers experience some degree of PND and up to 5 per cent are severely affected.

Dysthymia
Dysthymia involves persistent low mood with symptoms that are less severe or invasive than those experiences in depression. While the symptoms for this condition are less disabling and

less severe and therefore do not meet the diagnosis of a major depression, they will still prevent the person from feeling good about themselves and they may affect some functioning. The lower level symptoms of dysthymia may be experienced for a longer period, approximately two years (Davison & Neale, 2001).

Depression and the elderly

Depression is the most common mental illness in old people and the second most common single underlying cause for all GP consultations for people over 70 years of age. The pattern of depression is similar for elderly people and they suffer the same symptoms, however, there are different patterns of symptom awareness – the elderly often do not complain of low mood, as the physical manifestation of depression may be more obvious. Anxiety is a common feature of depression in the elderly often linked to forgetfulness and confusion and therefore a fear of dementia.

Depression and physical illness

Depression is very common in chronic physical illness but it is often undiagnosed, and therefore left untreated, as it is masked by the symptoms and effects of the physical condition. NIMH estimates that for individuals diagnosed with specific conditions, the levels of depression in specific illness is as follows:

- Cancer: 25 per cent
- Strokes: 10–27 per cent
- Heart attacks: 1 in 3
- HIV: 1 in 3
- Parkinson's disease: 50 per cent
- Eating disorders: 50–75 per cent

- Substance use: 27 per cent
- Diabetes: 8.5–28 per cent

In addition, depression may be triggered by a viral infection such as glandular fever (infectious mononucleosis) or flu (influenza) and in hypothyroidism, hypertension and degenerative disorders such as multiple sclerosis. It may also be a side effect of some medication.

DIAGNOSIS

The standard diagnosis for depression is based on the following criteria plus an interview with a clinician. However, there are several organic conditions that present with depressive symptoms so a differential diagnosis (weighing the probability of one condition versus others) may be necessary to exclude these.

Older classifications of depression such as endogenous-reactive (occurring as a result of stress or other traumatic life event) depression are no longer used, as evidence from stressful life-event research shows almost all episodes of depression are preceded by stressful life events and are therefore reactive. Cantopher (2003:6) suggests that depression caused by stressful events and circumstances is the most common cause.

Depression is diagnosed if there are symptoms present that interfere with daily functioning, accompanied by a low mood for a minimum of two weeks.

For ease, many GPs use the Patient Health Questionnaire 9 (PHQ-9) or the Hospital Anxiety and Depression Scale (HADS) to diagnose and monitor depression in primary care. These simple questionnaires are validated for use in primary health care settings and suggest a range of treatment options.

Diagnostic criteria

Criteria A: Five or more of the following present during a two-week period, nearly every day, and represent a change from previous functioning. At least one of the symptoms must be either I depressed mood or 2 loss of interest or pleasure.

A(1) Depressed mood (can be irritable mood in children/adolescents)

A(2) Markedly diminished interest or pleasure in all, or almost all, activity

A(3) Significant weight loss or weight gain when not dieting

A(4) Insomnia or hypersomnia

A(5) Psychomotor agitation or retardation

A(6) Fatigue or loss of energy

A(7) Feelings of worthless or excessive or inappropriate guilt

A(8) Diminished ability to think or concentrate

A(9) Recurrent thoughts of death, recurrent suicide ideation without a specific plan or a suicidal attempt or a specific plan for committing suicide

Criteria B: Symptoms are not better accounted for by a mood disorder due to a general medical condition, a substance-induced mood disorder, or bereavement (normal reaction to death of a loved one).

Criteria C: Symptoms are not better accounted for by a psychotic disorder (for example schizoaffective disorder).

CAUSES

There are various theories regarding the causes of depression, areas of which include:

- Biological (brain chemistry)
- Genetic disposition (heredity)
- Environmental and social factors (stress, relationship problems, illness, bereavement, loss of job, life transitions, etc.)
- Psychoanalytic (early developmental experiences)
- Cognitive-behavioural (thinking patterns)
- Humanistic (low self-worth)
- Family systems (relationships and roles within the family)

Depression is more likely if another family member has experienced depression, although there is no evidence to indicate that a specific genetic link exists. An alternative theory is that families tend to occupy similar environments and share learned behaviour, beliefs and ways of dealing with emotions and situations, so depression may be a learned response (nurture), rather than a genetic response (nature).

Gender

Depression is generally reported to be more common in women, than in men. However, this may be due to cultural and social factors ('big boys don't cry') that cause men to hide their more vulnerable feelings or mask and suppress these feelings with alcohol or other substances or behaviours. Likewise, women may learn to suppress anger ('women don't get angry').

Environmental and social factors

Stress, relationship problems, illness, bereavement, loss of a job, life transitions, giving birth, getting divorced, etc. are all lifestyle factors that have the potential to contribute to feelings of depression.

Chemical

There is some evidence that suggests an imbalance of the chemicals in the brain that send and receive messages – the neurotransmitters (e.g. serotonin and norepinephrine) – contribute to depression. This can usually be corrected by medication, which rebalances and increases the concentration of these chemicals so that the messages in the brain can occur more efficiently. Other lifestyle factors that may affect the chemical balance include diet, alcohol, drugs and physical activity and inactivity.

Early developmental experiences

Early life experiences, such as experiencing significant loss (the death of a parent or caregiver) may contribute to depression at that time or in later life, when it is triggered by an experience that evokes similar feelings (abandonment, loss, rejection, etc.) Alternatively, growing up with a parent, caregiver or teacher who is constantly critical or ridiculing can contribute to a low self-worth that contributes to depression. Abuse (verbal, physical, emotional, sexual or neglect) can also lead to depression and other mental health problems (e.g. substance abuse, eating disorders).

Attachment theory suggests that a 'lack of attachment' to a significant person during the early years can also cause long-term depression later in life. The theory assumes that we are all born as 'social' beings with a need to develop intimate relationships. These relationships start at birth, usually with our mothers (or other significant other, such as a grandparent). As a baby, we cry out for our needs to be met. In a healthy relationship, our mothers respond with the right amount of attention. From this secure base, we explore our world knowing that we could come back to our mother and be greeted with affection. An insecurely attached child can be very clingy, afraid to explore his/her world and angry with his/her mother. Research has now shown that an insecurely attached child quite often has mental ill-health repercussions later in life.

However, attachment theorists (Winnicott) also suggests that there is no such thing as the ideal parent and that most parents will do the best they can with the resources they have available. They suggest that being 'good enough' is good enough for us to develop a healthy mental well-being.

Self-worth

People with chronically low self-esteem or self-worth are more at risk of depression than persons with a more realistic sense of esteem and self-value. A person's perceived 'self-worth' will be influenced by early developmental experiences and other experiences throughout their life span.

Thinking patterns

Constant negative thinking, such as 'this is terrible, it is awful, it is dreadful, life sucks, I'm hopeless, etc.' have the potential to create a downward spiralling mood that can contribute to depression. The way we think may be linked to early developmental experiences and experiences within the family (learned thinking) and other life experiences.

Repressed or suppressed emotions

Some theories suggest that depression is caused by feelings or emotions that are not expressed; these may include sadness, anger, guilt, shame, loneliness, etc. In fact, any feeling that is not expressed can be turned inwards against the self. It is suggested by some theorists that depression is anger turned inward against the self, which may contribute to other problems, such as self-harm, risk-taking behaviour, substance abuse and even suicide.

Some feelings, when vented outwardly in an inappropriate way (anger), may alienate others. However, all emotions need expression, so talking therapies and self-help tools, such as letter writing or painting, can be a useful vent for pent-up feelings.

As Strock (2000) suggests, a combination of these factors can contribute to the onset of depression and later episodes may be 'precipitated by only mild stresses or none at all'.

TREATMENTS
GP

The first line of any treatment plan is to seek diagnosis from a GP. Asking for help is not a sign of weakness; it is an essential first step to recovery. Most GPs will recommend that if medication is prescribed, it should be accompanied with self-help strategies and/or therapy or counselling. The strategies recommended will depend on the severity of the depression and the individual circumstances.

Drugs and medications

As depression is diagnosed using a medical model of criteria, the most common treatment is pharmacological. There are many drugs used to treat depression and as new ones are coming on to the market regularly, it is important to keep up to date with names and side effects. Instructors working with individuals with mental health problems must take the side effects of any prescribed medication into account as they can have a profound effect on exercise participation, ability and adherence. It may be necessary to consult the doctor or Community Psychiatric Nurse (CPN) to get the full prescription of a client and it is essential to be aware of timings and dosages of drugs.

Most drugs in this group have side effects that start to occur immediately and these can be very troublesome. Unfortunately, the benefits of the drug may take weeks or even months to take effect, which means that many people stop taking them without medical guidance. On the plus side, side effects usually wear off or are better tolerated after a few weeks when the benefits become established.

Antidepressants

There are several types of antidepressant medication used to treat the symptoms of moderate and severe depression. They can be prescribed to treat mild depression, but other forms of treatment may be used initially. They are intended as a short-term intervention to ameliorate the symptoms of the condition while longer-term treatment such as therapy is put into place.

Antidepressants block the receptors responsible for the reuptake or breakdown of certain chemicals, principally noradrenalin and serotonin, which stimulate the brain cells and affect mood. Reduced levels of these chemicals occur in depression so, by blocking the receptors, these drugs help to maintain higher levels in the brain and lead to a reduction in depressive symptoms.

It should be noted that they are not 'happy' pills; rather they are designed to stop the individual feeling low so that energy and motivation improves to aids recovery.

Table 2.1	Overview of antidepressant drugs
Information	**Side effects**
Tricyclic antidepressants (TCAs): e.g. Amitriptyline, Dosulepin, Imipramine	
Introduced in the 1950s, TCAs are still used to treat depression, although they can take up to several weeks to work. Some TCAs have a sedative effect so may be prescribed to patients who are also anxious and agitated.	Sedation, blurred vision, arrhythmias (irregular heartbeat), tachycardia (increased heart rate), syncope (transient loss of consciousness), sweating, tremor, behavioural disturbances, hypomania, mania, weight gain (or loss) convulsions, movement disorders, urinary retention, constipation, dry mouth, confusion, postural hypotension.
Selective serotonin reuptake inhibitors (SSRIs): e.g. Fluoxetine (Prozac), Citalopram, Paroxetine (Seroxat)	
Introduced in the 1980s, SSRIs are hailed by many doctors as the biggest single drug breakthrough in modern times. Side effects are fewer and they are less sedative than TCAs. SSRIs appear to be better tolerated than many other types of antidepressants.	Common: Gastro-intestinal disorders, anorexia with weight loss (or gain), angioedema, arthralgia and myalgia, nervousness, anxiety, headache, insomnia, tremor, dizziness, asthenia (weakness, lack of energy), drowsiness, sweating, movement disorders, visual disturbances and hypomania or mania.
Monoamine oxidase inhibitors (MAOIs) and reversible inhibitors of monoamine oxidase (RIMAs) e.g. Moclobemide, Isocarboxazid	
Used when other treatments have been unsuccessful, not as a first line treatment due to the reaction with tyramine contained in some foods (e.g. processed meats, pork, fermented food, chocolate, alcohol, cheese, yoghurt, tofu, avocado, some fruits, yeast, Brazil nuts, coconut). NB: These foods are also linked to migraine.	Tyramine: Muscle spasms, headache or vomiting, a sudden potentially fatal rise in blood pressure. General: Sleep disturbance, dizziness, gastrointestinal disorders, headache, restlessness, agitation, oedema, paraesthesia and confusion, dry mouth, urinary retention and confusion, postural hypotension.
Atypical antidepressants: Venlafaxine	
Selective serotonin and noradrenalin reuptake inhibitor (SNRIs). Noradrenergic and selective serotonergic acting drugs (NaSSAs). Noradrenalin reuptake inhibitors (NRIs).	Gastro-intestinal disturbances, dizziness, insomnia, drowsiness, sweating, weight changes, hypertension, palpitation, arthralgia, myalgia, light-headedness, vertigo, postural hypotension, tachycardia and paraesthesia.

It should be noted that the therapeutic effects of these medications may not be felt for up to eight weeks but side effects are experienced immediately, which may result in the patient giving up the medication too soon.

Antidepressants are helpful as part of a treatment plan because they manage the symptoms. However, they will not treat the **cause** of the depression so it is recommended that medication be taken alongside lifestyle changes or therapy. After three months of treatment, research shows that between 50 and 65 per cent of individuals improve if given an antidepressant (hence the need for medication to go hand in hand with self-help/therapy/counselling). Without any treatment, most depressions will get better after about eight months, however if a patient stops taking the medication before eight or nine months is up, the symptoms of depression are more likely to return. The current recommendation is that it is best to continue to take antidepressants for at least six months after the person starts to feel better. If they have had two or more attacks of depression then treatment should be continued for at least two years. Antidepressants are not addictive although there may be some withdrawal symptoms when discontinuing use.

Anti-anxiety drugs or sedatives

These are sometimes prescribed alongside antidepressants to assist with anxiety and promote sleeping. They are not effective for treating a depressive disorder if taken alone (Strock, 2000). The most commonly used is the benzodiazepine (BDZ) group. They produce effective short-term benefits but are highly addictive and therefore not recommended for long-term use. (See page 35 for more information on these medications.)

Antidepressants and exercise

Once the drug is established the side effects are likely to reduce but there may still be exercise implications. Any cardiac side effects, including increased blood pressure, postural hypotension, tachycardia, arrhythmias, syncope and known ECG changes need full medical clearance before exercise participation.

The possible side effects of some medication such as joint pain (arthralgia) or muscle pain (myalgia) will limit intensity and duration of exercise and may affect exercise choice while paraesthesia (the sensation of pricking, burning or numbness in the nerves) and peripheral nerve damage may restrict the ability to hold or grip equipment so alternatives must be considered.

If an individual experiences any balance issues or dizziness, including postural or orthostatic hypotension, seated exercise may be advised, or the patient should avoid any sudden or frequent changes in position that may increase the risk of falling.

While weight gain may not prevent exercise, it may cause the individual to feel self-conscious or have a negative body image. This is particularly true in those who maintained a healthy weight and body shape before the condition arose.

NB: Most of the medicines in the antidepressant group, particularly TCAs, may cause arrhythmias and convulsions, so an appropriate warm-up and cool down is essential.

Electroconvulsive therapy (ECT)

ECT was once a common treatment for a number of mental health problems, including major clinical depression that had not responded to other treatments. While its use has declined with the improvement in modern pharmacological treatments, it is still in use today, which raises some controversy (Bentall, 2010).

ECT involves sending a small electrical current through the brain to provoke a seizure, similar to 'resetting' a computer. Three quarters of patients treated with ECT show a definite improvement and many consider it the most effective treatment option for them. There were 12,800 administrations of (ECT) in England in the period January to March 2002 compared to 16,500 in January to March 1999 (DoH, 2003). Concerns exist about the long-term effects and involuntary use; figures from the DoH state that 60 per cent of the 600 patients treated with ECT in 2002 while formally detained did not consent to treatment. However, 73 per cent of patients receiving ECT were not formally detained under the Mental Health Act.

The most common side effects of ECT are headache, stiffness and confusion. Temporary memory loss on awakening from the treatment is also common and can be permanent in some cases. ECT may also cause spasms during treatment and there may be temporary numbness in the fingers and the toes.

Psychological therapies (psychotherapy)
Cognitive behavioural therapy (CBT)
CBT is one of the most effective types of treatment for anxiety and depression, possibly improving the symptoms of over half of those diagnosed with the condition. CBT focuses on helping to identify unhelpful and unrealistic thoughts and beliefs (cognitions) and behaviour patterns. Strategies to replace these with more positive and helpful thoughts and behaviours are discussed and put into practice. Unlike many forms of therapy, CBT focuses on the present, not the past and teaches

new skills and coping strategies to help respond positively to situations that would normally cause anxiety and depression. The recent government strategy paper 'No health without mental health' (2011) cites the potential use of CBT as part of the treatment plan to achieve the 6 objectives listed. Some GPs already work in collaboration with counsellors in training and provide them with supervised work placements, which enable the counsellor to gain the required counselling hours to achieve BACP (British Association of Counselling and Psychotherapy) accreditation, which cements their qualification.

The National Institute for Health and Clinical Excellence (NICE) recommends a total of 16–20 hours of CBT, usually in one- to two-hour long weekly sessions.

Psychodynamic
Psychodynamic treatments tend to work at deeper levels to resolve inner conflicts and are usually only introduced when the depression has significantly improved. This is a longer term therapy and is usually only available through private practice and is often quite expensive.

Interpersonal therapy (IPT)/problem-solving therapy
IPT focuses on relationships with other people and on problems such as difficulties with communication or coping with bereavement. There is some evidence that IPT can be as effective as medication or CBT, but more research is needed.

Humanistic
Humanistic or person-centred approaches focus on listening and building an empathic,

non-judgmental, congruent relationship where the individual can discuss their problems. This is usually a longer term therapy and is usually only available through private practice. However, all other therapies will have humanistic values and the core conditions at the heart of their practice.

Group therapy

This is a useful form of therapy for some people, as talking though common problems helps them realise they are not alone and is a useful way to get support and advice. It is often recommended for people with OCD or eating disorders, and children and young people with mild depression. Group therapy may take the form of guided self help groups which may be available through some mental health services. It may also take the form of private therapy to work with families who are experiencing difficulties.

NB: The British Association of Counselling and Psychotherapy provide a list of accredited counsellors and provide an ethical framework to inform the practice of all members.

Self-help/bibliotherapy

There is a wide range of self-help books and strategies to assist with personal management of depression.

Alternative treatments
St John's Wort

This herbal treatment is often taken for depression, however, although there is some evidence that it may be of benefit when treating mild or moderate depression, it is not widely used. The main reason for this is the variation in quality and quantity of brands and batches, making its effects uncertain (Linde et al. 2008). St. John's Wort may also cause serious problems when used in conjunction with other medications such as anticonvulsants, anti-coagulants, antidepressants and the contraceptive pill and it can cause photosensitivity.

Acupuncture

The WHO lists depression among the conditions for which acupuncture is effective. However, there is a lack of reliable evidence to prove it can work for depression (Smith et al., 2010).

Homeopathy

This complementary system of medicine treats the whole person, taking into account physical and psychological type as well as disease symptoms. One of its main principles is that 'Like cures like', in other words the symptoms of an illness caused by a substance will be cured by the same substance given in homoeopathic form. However, there is very little reliable evidence into the effects on depression so its use cannot be validated (Pilkington et al., 2005).

Diet

Depressive symptoms can be exacerbated by nutritional deficiencies so good nutrition is important and a well-balanced and unprocessed diet is recommended. Cutting back on stimulants such as caffeine and tobacco, and reducing the use of depressants including alcohol, is advised and quitting smoking is recommended.

Aromatherapy

Aromas may lower stress levels, affect mood and even change perceptions of pain. Research is currently (2011) being done at University of Wales Institute, Cardiff (UWIC) into whether aromatherapy is a benefit for individuals with depression. For more information visit www. journeysonline.co.uk.

Exercise as therapy

The use of exercise as an initial treatment for mild depression and anxiety, and as an adjunct to other treatments in mild and moderate cases, is increasing and there is increasing research and evidence to recommend the use of exercise and activity in the treatment of mild to moderate depression (Biddle et al., 2000; Halliwell, 2005). NICE recently made the recommendation that persons with depression (mild to moderate) should be advised of the benefits of following a structured and supervised exercise programme of typically up to three sessions per week of moderate duration (45 minutes to 1 hour) for between 10–14 weeks (NICE, 2009). Although self-directed increases in activity and exercise are beneficial, the motivation to start and to keep going may be more of a problem. As a result, it is increasingly common for people with mental health problems to be referred by a health care provider to an appropriate scheme for exercise. Exercise on referral is one type of intervention used to promote exercise and physical activity to benefit health and there are a range of initiatives throughout the UK (Halliwell, 2005).

Research by the mental health organisation MIND showed that 58 per cent of people with mental health problems did not know that GPs can prescribe exercise sessions and activities while 42 per cent claimed they did know. The biggest barriers preventing those with mental health problems from taking part in physical exercise were motivation problems (39 per cent), the cost of doing sporting activities (33 per cent) and lack of confidence (31 per cent). These can be partly addressed by the motivational and financial support provided by an exercise referral scheme. Interestingly 59 per cent of the public stated that they thought exercise could help prevent people from developing mental health problems such as depression and anxiety – yet only 30 per cent are active at a level beneficial for health.

The Mental Health Foundation report 'Up and Running' (2005) examined some of the reasons for a lack of referral for exercise that exist in the medical profession. It concluded that a lack of awareness of the benefits of exercise and availability of suitable referral schemes among GPs may be one of the biggest barriers to recommendation. At the time the report was published only 1 per cent of GPs referred patients with mental health problems for exercise, yet paradoxically 42 per cent would try exercise as a treatment option if they themselves became depressed.

Exercise recommendations for depressive disorders

The specific type and amount of exercise recommended is dependent on a number of factors. Exercise professionals working with this population should conduct a detailed screening assessment and work with other health care professionals, if appropriate and if the client agrees, to identify ways of supporting the person. The severity of the condition is a primary consideration as some clients with depression are de-motivated and even regular daily activities, such as housework, are too much. In these instances, it may be worth the patient seeking counselling support to discuss and learn to manage the thoughts and feelings that contribute to this state prior to embarking on an exercise programme.

Other considerations include the side effects specific medications can have on exercise and the treatments of any other coexisting medical conditions (which can be varied). It may be that depression occurs in response to another medical condition (rheumatoid arthritis, heart disease, cancer) in which case the exercise and activity plan would need to be different than if depression presented as an isolated condition. Each of these issues should be considered prior to making any exercise prescription or recommendations.

As a guideline, Durstine & Moore (2003:317) recommend following the ACSM prescription for the general population with a more conservative approach in relation to intensity, as inactivity, high body fat and low self-esteem may be more common in this population. Age, fitness and current activity levels will also affect the exercise recommended. The Active for Health prescription (DoH, 1996 and 2005) can be offered as a preliminary target guideline for building activity to a level that can assist with the maintenance of health and promote general feelings of well-being.

The appropriateness of specific types of activity will be dependent on the individual and the existence of other medical conditions (obesity, high blood pressure, etc.). For example, an overweight individual would be advised to perform lower impact and non-weight bearing activities, whereas, an individual with osteoporosis or osteoarthritis would need to follow the specific guidelines that account for their individual conditions.

- **Cardiovascular** exercise can contribute to a 'feel good factor' (release of endorphins), which can motivate the individual to take on other activities.
- **Muscular strength and endurance** activities assist with muscle tone and shape, which can contribute to increased physical self-esteem.
- **Flexibility and mobility** exercises assist with efficiency of movement, making daily tasks easier. Stretching also assists with relaxation and can improve posture, which in turn can have an impact on increasing confidence.

Cardiovascular	Muscle fitness	Flexibility	Functional
• 3–5 days a week • RPE 11–14 (on 6–20 scale) • 20–30 minutes • Large muscles, walk, run, swim, cycle (Adapted from Durstine & Moore, 2003:317)	• 2 days a week • 1–2 sets • 8–12 repetitions • 50–70 per cent of 1RM • Whole body approach	• 5 days a week • To point of mild discomfort • 20–60 seconds • Whole body approach	• Promote ADL daily • Activity related to daily living • 30 minutes • Walking • Gardening • Housework

Figure 2.1 ACSM Exercise Guidelines for Depression

Exercise implications

Low levels of motivation will require sensitivity and patience on the part of the exercise professional. When people feel depressed, they are often unmotivated to do housework or other everyday tasks that were previously undertaken. A supportive and encouraging and empathic approach is essential.

Energy levels may also be low and the person may feel tired a lot of the time, therefore intensity needs to be lowered, perhaps through including rests in the session or taking an accumulative approach to the activity. The positive benefits of exercise need to be reinforced and the person must be praised for small efforts, which can make a big difference to their overall health.

Medication can have an effect on heart rate, blood pressure, energy levels and may contribute to weight gain. All of these side effects must be accounted for prior to recommending any specific exercise programme.

Enjoyment and fun should be incorporated into the activity and where possible socialisation, for example, group exercise, where participants can encourage and support each other. The inclusion of specific relaxation techniques that the person can practice at home is useful for managing anxiety. Frequency, intensity, time, type of activity will be determined by other individual factors already discussed.

ANXIETY RELATED DISORDERS

Anxiety is an unpleasant emotional state causing symptoms of subjective fear, emotional and/or physical discomfort and physiological effects. Anxiety is more common in women than men and typical onset is in early adult life (DSM).

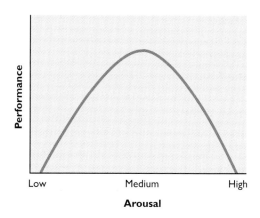

Figure 2.2 Yerkes-Dodson law

It is well documented that performance increases with physiological or mental arousal, but this only occurs up to a point. When levels of arousal or stress become too high, performance decreases. Known as the Yerkes-Dodson law, after Robert Yerkes and John Dodson who first developed the theory in 1908, it is demonstrated by the curve shown in figure 2.2, which shows that we function better in the middle of the curve with medium arousal rather than with low or high levels of arousal.

PREVALENCE

There are a number of anxiety disorders affecting around 9 per cent of the population at any one time. The most common are generalised anxiety disorders (2–6 per cent of the population), panic disorders (up to 5 per cent of the population) and phobic disorders. Long-term anxiety can lead to obsessive-compulsive disorder (OCD), which is estimated to affect at least 2–3 per cent of the population (Semple, 2005).

CAUSES

There is no specific, identifiable cause of anxiety, however it often occurs co-morbidly with other mental health disorders such as depression or through alcohol or substance abuse. Other potential causes include an imbalance of certain chemicals in the brain, particularly serotonin and noradrenalin, or suffering with hypoglycaemia or some thyroid disorders. However, anxiety is likely to be due to a combination of causes, genetic influences, environment, life experiences and circumstances and biological factors and it may not be possible to isolate an overall cause.

TYPES OF ANXIETY DISORDERS
Generalised anxiety disorder

The psychological effects of anxiety include a sense of impending threat or dread or fear of death out of proportion to an existent threat. Other symptoms of anxiety disorders include restlessness, feeling on edge, difficulty concentrating or being easily distracted, irritability, impatience, constant vigilance and catastrophising.

The physical symptoms of anxiety can cause significant distress and affect everyday life and function. These include lethargy, dizziness, palpitations, muscle aches, excessive perspiration, shortness of breath, pins and needles, gastrointestinal problems, headache and/or migraine, excessive thirst, frequent urination, menstrual problems, difficulty in falling or staying asleep. It is also common to worry about events that are improbable or out of the person's control.

Most people have experienced anxiety at some time, often before an isolated event such as an examination, public speaking or interview but for others, with trait anxiety, that is the predisposition to become anxious in certain situations, this becomes pervasive and when one situation is over, another becomes the trigger for the anxiety.

Individuals with phobic disorder or panic disorder will know the trigger for their anxious state and usually go to great lengths to avoid it. However, individuals with generalised anxiety disorder may not know the exact cause of their anxiousness.

Phobias

Davison & Neale (2001:128) describe a phobia as a: 'Disrupting fear and avoidance that is out of proportion to the danger posed by the feared object/situation and which is recognised by the person as groundless'. Phobias can severely restrict life and trigger a panic attack and there is an 80 per cent risk of developing another psychiatric disorder (DSM-IV-TR). While there may be a specific phobic trigger, it is not necessarily dangerous or threatening, it is the feelings that they induce that are the problem.

There are many identified phobias from spiders (arachnophobia) to flying (aviophobia), to blood (haemophobia). Causes are many and include the displacement of an unconscious conflict, learned behaviour or a negative experience. It is thought that poor life experiences can make people more vulnerable to developing a phobia and they are often seen in adults who were brought up by over-anxious parents.

The most frequently encountered phobia is agoraphobia (60 per cent of those with a phobia) which is a fear of being in a situation from which there is no escape. This often leads to a socially isolated life based in, or very close to, the home.

Treatment is usually in the form of a talking therapy or behaviour therapy, also known as exposure therapy which involves controlled, gradual exposure to the phobic trigger, and medication such as benzodiazepines (tranquilisers) may be used to control the short-term effects of the phobia.

Social phobia (social anxiety disorder)

Social phobia is a marked and persistent fear of social or performance situations in which discomfort or embarrassment may occur, particularly involving 'performance' such as public speaking. This leads to fear of others noticing or looking at the person and can involve a fear of eating or drinking in public. It results in high levels of anxiety and/or panic attacks and may lead to withdrawal from social life.

Around 1–2 per cent of men and 2–3 per cent of women will develop a social phobia (DSM-IV-TR) and it is increasingly common in adolescents, particularly around the time of transfer to secondary school.

Treatment includes social skills training, exposure therapy or cognitive therapy and medication may be used to control the symptoms of anxiety or panic.

Obsessive-compulsive disorder (OCD)

Characterised by unwelcome, persistent, recurrent thoughts, ideas, fears, compulsions, images or impulses that are uncomfortable, intrusive or senseless, OCD is a common feature of depression and anxiety. It can be very time consuming with repetitive behaviour taking up at least 1 hour of the day, sometimes up to 6 hours or more that can have a profound effect on daily life.

Onset is usually in adolescence and more common where another family member also has OCD. Tourette's syndrome and tics are also common family traits that co-exist with OCD.

OCD is estimated to affect 1 in 50 people but is likely to affect many more who are adept at hiding the condition.

Recent research has shown a link between functional abnormalities in the brain as well as abnormalities of neurotransmitters, particularly serotonin and the development of OCD (DSM-IV, 2007, Semple 2005). This theory is still in development, however it may provide an insight into why the condition develops in some people and not others. It is also suggested that it may be a defensive mechanism against sadistic or aggressive fantastical thoughts that can be replaced by filling the mind with obsessive thoughts instead (Semple, 2005).

Treatment involves counselling and psychotherapy, CBT, medication and residential treatments, often with other people with OCD. In severe cases, neurosurgery has been a treatment option, although thankfully this is very rare and its use is controversial (Bentall, 2010).

Table 2.1	Most common traits in OCD	
Most common obsessions	**Most common compulsions**	
Fear of contamination	Cleaning and washing	
Fear of causing harm	Checking	
Fear of mistakes	Touching	
Fear of unacceptable behaviour	Arranging and organising	
Need for symmetry or exactness	Collecting and hoarding	
Excessive doubt	Counting and repeating	

Panic attacks

Panic attacks are characterised by a sudden and overwhelming sense of fear or terror, which brings on panic and apprehension. They can occur in conjunction with both anxiety and depressive disorders and often occur in situations that are not dangerous but which appear threatening to the individual. They can be spontaneous (sudden) or situational (occurring in similar situations to previous attacks) when there is a pattern of repeated attacks it is referred to as panic disorder.

Panic attacks may be triggered by a variety of situations or emotions from public speaking to coming face to face with a phobic trigger. The person may experience laboured breathing, a choking sensation, hyperventilation, palpitations, sweating, giddiness and nausea. More severe symptoms such as derealisation (sense of unreality), depersonalisation (a sense of watching oneself act without any control over actions), fear of dying, fear of going 'crazy' or of losing control can have a significant effect on an individual both during an attack or in everyday life due to the fear of an attack.

In more severe cases medical intervention such as rapid tranquilisation may be necessary and ongoing treatment in the form of antidepressants, benzodiazepines or anxiolytics may be helpful. CBT and relaxation techniques such as learning to breathe calmly when feeling an attack coming on can reduce most of the physical symptoms and bring back a state of calm.

TREATMENT FOR ANXIETY DISORDERS
Medication
Anxiolytic (anti-anxiety) drugs

Anxiolytic drugs are prescribed in the short term to treat the symptoms and effects of anxiety and may also be used to treat anxiety disorders. They do not normally affect the underlying causes of anxiety, hence the short-term use. There are two main groups: anxiolytics and hypnotics.

Benzodiazepines (BZDs), classified as minor tranquilisers (although their side effects such as sedation can be major), have a relatively rapid effect, while the non-benzodiazepines, including buspirone (a 5-hydroxytryptamine or serotonin receptor agonist) are less sedative but take several weeks to have an effect.

The older barbiturate group which includes amylobarbitone, methyl pnenobarbitone and phenobarbitone, is rarely used to treat anxiety today but is still in use as a treatment for insomnia. Additionally, beta-blockers, more commonly used to treat hypertension may be used to alleviate the symptoms and effects of anxiety such as increased heart rate, sweating and shaking by reducing the nervous system responses to stress, while SSRIs or SNRIs (see Depression, page 26) may be to treat long-term or non-responsive anxiety.

Antihistamines, normally used to treat allergic reactions, are used in the short-term treatment of anxiety. They work by calming the brain, thereby reducing the level of perceived anxiety, but are only effective when used for short periods.

Table 2.2	Overview of anxiolytic drugs
Information	**Side effects**
Anxiolytics and hypnotics (benzodiazepines (BZDs), barbiturates and 'Z' drugs)	
These reduce physical symptoms of anxiety, promote relaxation and have a sedative effect. They are also a muscle relaxant.	Daytime drowsiness, dizziness, unsteadiness, muscle weakness, reduced alertness, confusion, blurred vision and slower reactions.
Antidepressants (tricyclics)	
Introduced in the 1950s, TCAs are still used to treat depression, although they can take up to several weeks to work. Some TCAs have a sedative effect so may be prescribed to patients who are also anxious and agitated.	Sedation, blurred vision, arrhythmias, ECG changes, syncope (transient loss of consciousness), tachycardia, sweating, tremor, behavioural disturbances, hypomania, mania, weight gain (or weight loss), convulsions, movement disorders, urinary retention, constipation, dry mouth, confusion, postural hypotension.
5-HT$_{1A}$ agonists – buspirone	
Lacks the cognitive and sedative effects and the dependence of BZDs, however those used to the sedative effects of BZDs may not find it effective.	Nausea, dizziness, headache, nervousness, light-headedness and excitement. Caution: May affect driving or machine operation.
Beta-blockers	
Depress the action of the sympathetic nervous system and reduce the physical symptoms of anxiety such as tachycardia, muscle tension and agitation.	Hypotension, bradycardia, fatigue SOB/wheezing, GI disturbances, lethargy, sleep disturbance, peripheral vasoconstriction, cold extremities, leg pain, cramps.
Antihistamines – hydroxyzine	
These have a calming effect on the brain, reducing anxiety.	Drowsiness, dizziness, blurred vision, headache, dry mouth.

Anxiolytic medications and exercise

The side effect of BZDs such as drowsiness, dizziness and ataxia (a neurological disorder affecting balance, speech and coordination) necessitate careful exercise choice to avoid sudden or frequent changes in direction, complex moves or positions requiring good balance and stability. The length and intensity of the session will need consideration to avoid fatigue. The muscle-relaxing effects of this drug necessitate caution when stretching to avoid over-lengthening the muscle or hyperextension of the joint.

Buspirone and hydroxyzine affect motor skills, necessitating that movements be simple with ample time for rehearsal or changes in position or direction. Avoid complex movements or combinations due to reduced motor skills and the possibility of nervousness or agitation. Aim to promote a sense of mastery and achievement.

Beta-blockers have many exercise implications to consider. The blunting effect on heart rate will preclude the use of heart rate monitoring, so use a more subjective rating of effort such as Rating of Perceived Exertion (RPE) instead. Peripheral vasoconstriction (constriction of the blood vessels outside the core of the body) can lead to leg aches and cramps and an accumulation of lactic acid leading to acute and chronic muscle soreness. Bronchospasms, tiredness and lethargy may reduce exercise tolerance while movement quality may deteriorate.

Talking treatments

Initially talking treatments are used to treat anxiety. There are many forms of this type of therapy and some are discussed in the section on depression (see page 28).

CBT

CBT is one of the most effective types of treatment for anxiety, possibly improving the symptoms of over half of those diagnosed with the condition. The focus of CBT is on helping to identify unhelpful and unrealistic thoughts and beliefs (cognitions) and behaviour patterns. Strategies to replace these with more positive and helpful thoughts and behaviours are identified and put into practice.

Unlike many forms of therapy, CBT focuses on the present, not the past and teaches new skills and coping strategies to help respond positively to situations that would normally cause anxiety. NICE recommends a total of 16–20 hours of CBT, usually in one- to two-hour long weekly sessions.

Exposure therapy

This is used to treat phobias through gradual exposure to the trigger and teaching strategies to prevent the 'panic' response.

Group therapy

Group therapy is a useful form of therapy for OCD, as talking though common compulsions and obsessions helps patients to realise they are not alone and is a useful way to get support and advice.

Diet

Diet has an important role in mental health. A healthy, varied and balanced diet will provide the necessary nutrients for development and repair is a key factor in positive mental health. The Royal College of Psychiatrists publish a booklet, *Eating Well*, which covers basic healthy nutritional guidelines and also includes more specific recommendations for mental health conditions such as schizophrenia and mood disorders. Visit www.rcpsych.ac.uk/mentalhealthinfo/problems/nutrition for more information. Reducing intake of caffeine and alcohol and cutting down on (or preferably giving up) smoking may help to ease symptoms of anxiety as these substances all disrupt sleep and increase the heart rate. Smoking and alcohol are also known to worsen anxiety. Staying within the recommended guidelines (no more than 3–4 units of alcohol a day for men and 2–3 units a day for women, i.e. half a pint of ordinary strength lager, a pub measure (25ml) of spirits, or a small glass (125ml) of lower alcohol (11 per cent) wine) will also help.

Exercise

Exercise, in particular aerobic exercise, has a major role to play in alleviating the onset and symptoms of anxiety. There are strong links between regular activity and a reduction in trait anxiety, meaning that individuals are less likely to become anxious when in difficult situations (Morgan, 1997). An important consideration is the similarity of the effects of anxiety – faster heart rate, increased respiration rate, sweating and muscle tension – to the physiological response to exercise. Prepare your participants or clients for this by telling them what they can expect to happen or they may think they are having a panic attack, which can be distressing for all. On the plus side, as they experience the physiological effects of exercise, including increased heart rate, respiration, perspiration and muscle tension, in a controlled way, they may be able to consciously control or rationalise these symptoms when experiencing anxiety.

The standard guidelines apply – a minimum of 30 minutes of moderate exercise at least five days a week. This can be in the form of a brisk walk or swim or attending structured exercise sessions.

Relaxation, meditation and mindfulness

These are all useful tools to help with mental distress. Anything from relaxation and breathing exercises to tai chi, yoga or Pilates can help relieve tension and reduce anxiety and stress. Focusing on breathing offers a distraction and focus for the mind and the conscious action of slowing down the breath can contribute to the slowing down other physiological systems (e.g. slow down heart rate, which increases during panic and anxiety) that are out of conscious control. There is an increasing evidence base for the use of meditation and mindfulness practice (MHF 2010) for assisting with the management of anxiety, stress and depression. Mindfulness approaches help the person to concentrate on being 'in the moment' and staying aware of their body sensations, emotions and thoughts, without becoming stuck in any particular pattern (e.g. freeze-frame thinking

on one single negative or fearful thought). Instead the thoughts are encouraged to flow and be noticed as just thoughts. The way an individual thinks can have a direct impact on their feelings and emotions and the physical tension experienced by the body, so awareness of all of these brings control back to the individual; they can choose to change how they think, acknowledge and accept their physical and emotional experience and allow the sensations to pass, rather than remaining stuck.

STRESS

This is perhaps the most common of the stress and anxiety disorders and most people will experience excessive stress at some point in their life. A transient disorder usually occurring over a period of hours or days, stress is a reaction to an acute situation and will usually disperse once the situation, or 'threat', has ended. Those with trait anxiety may experience continuous stress reactions that become generalised anxiety disorder.

Generalised stress can be viewed as a psychological condition that will be influenced by an individual's perceived ability to balance the demands of their environment (work, relationships, health, etc.) with their internal and external coping resources (positive mental attitude, physical fitness, friends, family, finances, etc.).

Symptoms are similar to anxiety but may be more severe due to the acuteness of the situation. It is common for individuals to turn to alcohol or drugs to help them 'cope' with the situation and this may lead to an ongoing problem of substance dependency. Additionally, alcohol is a depressant so an increased intake may increase the likelihood of further mental health problems. Nicotine stimulates the sympathetic nervous system so increases the physiological effects of stress, which may be harmful in the long term.

If it is an isolated reaction the ending of the difficult situation will often alleviate the stress response. However, regular physical activity and exercise is recommended, and healthy eating patterns and a reduction in drinking, smoking or other substances will help both physically and psychologically.

Unhealthy stress and anxiety levels occur when the person feels unable to cope, and when they perceive a situation as applying an abnormal pressure, that taxes and exceeds their internal and external resources (Lawrence, 2005).

POST-TRAUMATIC STRESS DISORDER (PTSD)

PTSD is brought on by exposure to a stressful experience that is considered outside of the normal range of life events, for example, being the victim of or witnessing abuse, torture, accidents and/or disasters that involve death and traumatic human suffering. Someone experiencing PTSD will re-live the traumatic experience through repetitive thoughts or dreams, which cause the physical, mental and emotional responses brought on by the original event to be re-experienced. Learning to relax and re-framing the experience (e.g. reducing self-blame through CBT) are key methods of treatment. Medication is used to manage symptoms and social support can provide a sense of belonging and care that will ease the pain.

PREVALENCE

The MHF suggests:

- Over 12 million people visit their GP each year for mental health problems and most are diagnosed as suffering from anxiety and depression that is stress related (Daines et al., 1997).

The Occupational Health Statistics Bulletin (2002/3) indicates the following:

- Stress, anxiety and depression was reported as the second most commonly reported illness which individuals believed was caused or made worse by their current or past work.
- The prevalence of stress and related (mainly heart) conditions has increased and is double the level it was in 1990.
- In 2001/02 stress, depression or anxiety and musculoskeletal disorders accounted for the majority of work days lost.

The Health and Safety Executive (HSE) 2005 report cites research studies that indicate:

- Work-related stress, anxiety and depression account for 13 million reported lost working days per year.
- 254,000 people first became aware of work related stress, anxiety or depression in the previous 12 months.
- Over half a million individuals in Britain believed in 2003/4 that they were experiencing work-related stress that was making them ill.

CAUSES

There are numerous theories regarding the causes of stress, which include those listed for depression (brain chemistry, heredity, early developmental experiences, thinking patterns, etc.). A combination of the above and other social and environment factors, such as those listed on page 40, can trigger an individual to experience the stress response (fight or flight – see box).

- **Work:** Change of job, unemployment, redundancy, promotion, retirement
- **Relationships:** Marriage, divorce, birth of child, arguments with partner
- **Financial:** Mortgage, loans, debt, bankruptcy
- **Life events:** Death of relatives, partner or friends
- **Family:** Moving house, holidays, trouble with relatives
- **Health:** Changes in health status, diagnosis of a medical condition

Although most people may feel stressed or under pressure at some point in life, stress is not easy to define. It is a **psychological condition** that influences feelings and thoughts about and responses to different life events, demands and challenges in everyday life, strongly linked to the perception of ability to cope with these demands and experiences.

What is fight or flight?

Put simply, when we receive a stimulus or 'fright' our bodies prepare themselves either to attack – fight or retreat – flight. For example, if we come across a large fire our bodies prepare for flight to run away from it, while if we find a small fire we are more likely to experience a fight response and put it out. (Adapted from Lawrence, D and Bolitho, S. *Exercise Your Way to Health: Stress* (2011) A&C Black, UK.)

PERCEPTION

Stress can be perceived either positively or negatively; it is **positive**, as without stress there would be no life, no excitement or drive, yet too much or insufficient coping ability can have **negative** effects. There simply is no right or wrong way to see a situation – perception is simply the unique way that individuals experience life at a specific point in time. For example, being asked to speak in front of a group of people may for one person provide a challenge and a thrill or excitement (positive) whereas, the same offer may be experienced by another person as a terrifying ordeal that they need to avoid at all costs (negative).

DEMANDS AND RESOURCES

In potentially stressful situations, the more resources an individual has the more they perceive themselves as being able to cope.

Internal and external resources

Individuals may have **external** resources (e.g. friends, family, financial support, etc.) and **internal** resources (e.g. health, self-esteem, confidence and thinking patterns) and when these are in balance stress becomes manageable. If these resources are out of balance, stress can be overwhelming. Many individuals need help to see, and utilise, both their internal and external resources prior to and during times of stress and counselling and therapeutic interventions can help with this.

The givens

In life, there are many potential stressors over which an individual has no control – the 'givens'. How these are dealt with can have an impact upon stress levels so it is important to find a constructive solution to problems linked to 'givens'. In reality, while there may be small ways an individual can reduce their negative impact on the environment as a whole, it is more likely that they can have more of an impact in their own surroundings to help protect those near and dear. Given things are out of our control on a large scale, try to avoid allowing 'givens' to add more stress or worry to life.

THE STRESS RESPONSE

Humans have evolved substantitally since our hunter-gatherer days. Unfortunately, the way we respond to stressful situations has not evolved in the same way. To our earliest ancestors who had to deal with more physical demands, such as hunting for food or running from wild beasts, the fight or flight response was a great asset, but today it can result in internal accumulation of stress, as a great many of us are not achieving healthy targets of physical activity. This is one of the reasons why getting up and doing some exercise is so helpful for managing some of the signs and symptoms of stress. It uses your body's stress response and returns the body to a more balanced state.

WHAT IS GOING ON INSIDE?

As we now know, when we encounter a situation that makes us feel under pressure, or stressed, our body stimulates the fight or flight reaction, part of which is the release of chemicals such as adrenaline, noradrenaline and cortisol to help us deal with the threat. Unfortunately, we are not always in a position to fight or flee, for example, we are sat in a car, on a train, or at work, so these chemicals accumulate in the body.

The build up of adrenaline and noradrenaline over time increases heart rate, blood pressure and breathing rate. Blood supply is diverted from the digestive system to the muscles that tense up,

ready for action. Over time, the body remains in a perpetually 'semi-aroused' state that results in increased heart rate and blood pressure, muscle tension, poor digestion and a sense of edginess.

SIGNS AND SYMPTOMS OF STRESS

Some signs of stress are obvious and some are hidden. Figure 2.3 provides an example of some of the signs and symptoms of stress, however, many of these may come on over a period of time, which means they may not be immediately identified. Long-term exposure to stress can make us more susceptible to a range of health problems, including:

- High blood pressure
- High cholesterol
- Coronary heart disease
- Osteoporosis
- Depression
- Anxiety disorders
- Irritable bowel syndrome (IBS)
- Some cancers
- Alcohol related problems
- Eating disorders

Cortisol

Part of the stress reaction in the body is the release of fats and sugars into the bloodstream to provide instant energy for the fight or flight response. A build up of these can increase the risk of heart disease, as the combination of unused fats and sugar is nice and sticky and glues to the walls of the arteries. This reaction is triggered by increased levels of cortisol, a naturally occurring steroid hormone that can also have a negative effect on the skeleton, as it inhibits the cells that make bone and can lead to an increased risk of osteoporosis in individuals with chronic stress.

Physical	Mental	Emotional	Behavioural
Spots	Irrational thoughts	Sadness	Eat more or less
Muscle tension	Mental fatigue	Depressed	Drink more
Skin disorders	Procrastination	Angry	Smoke more
Chest pain	Low self-esteem	Fear	Swearing
Increased heart rate	Low self-worth	Panic/anxiety	Aggression, violence
Nervous indigestion	Inability to listen	Irritable	Risk taking
Breathing problems	Poor decision making	Bored	Change in libido
Yawning/sighing	Ego-centred	Lonely	Crying
Hypertension	Make mistakes	Jealousy	Crime
Abdominal pain	Accident prone	Resentment	Excessive talking
Sexual difficulties	Negative outlook	Helplessness	Foot tapping
Menstrual disorders	Blaming others or self	Loss of hope	Cannot sit still
Flatulence	Judgemental	Insecurity	Pick at skin/hair
Allergies	Critical of self and others	Frustration	Grind teeth
Hair loss		Tearful	Rapid eye movement
Dry mouth	Excessive self-criticism	Lethargy	Argumentative
Tension headaches		Unfocused	Nervous laughter

Figure 2.3 Signs and symptoms of stress

Cortisol also affects overall well-being by reducing the reactions to certain hormone signals in the body. This can result in lethargy and demotivation. It also leads to increased levels of chemicals such as insulin in the body resulting in insulin resistance, which can cause weight gain around the waist. Therefore, less stress or better coping strategies mean less cortisol and better well-being.

In instances where stress is prolonged, for example, being out of work for a long time or experiencing the effects of a debilitating condition (rheumatoid arthritis), the body has to find additional ways of coping. In these instances the hypothalamic-pituitary-adrenal (HPA) axis plays a role to ensure adequate energy needs to meet the extra demands on the body. It does this by stimulating the release of adrenocorticotropic hormone which in turn stimulates the release of cortisol. Cortisol enhances metabolic activity and raises blood glucose levels to provide energy when liver and muscle reserves have been used up.

TREATMENT
Medication
Medication can be used to assist with the management of anxiety and depressive symptoms. The medications prescribed for depression are used to treat specific stress related disorders, usually SSRIs for panic attacks and social phobias, tricyclics for general anxiety disorders (GAD) and panic attacks and benzodiazepines for general anxiety disorders and post-traumatic stress disorder (PTSD).

Self-help

There are numerous self-help books available to assist with the management of stress, anxiety and panic. Some self-help strategies (positive thinking, relaxation techniques, goal setting, time management, assertiveness) are discussed in *The Complete Guide to Exercising Away Stress* (Lawrence, 2005).

Breathing and relaxation

There is a tendency towards shallow and rapid breathing, using the upper thoracic or breathing from the chest (where the upper chest and shoulders lift and lower as we breathe). Poor breathing habits such as these can contribute to anxiety and panic. This type of breathing is also more common in people who are sedentary. Ideally, we should use the whole of the rib cage and abdomen when we breathe (diaphragm and abdominal breathing). Focusing on deeper and slower breathing can help to reduce the immediate and long-term effects of the fight and flight response and can help return the body to a more natural unstressed state.

Counselling and psychotherapy

Each of the therapies listed for depression are appropriate for exploring stress (see page 28). Therapists should be registered with either the British Association for Counselling and Therapy (BACP) or the United Kingdom Council for Psychotherapy (UKCP).

Alternative and complementary therapies

Nutrition, massage, reflexology and acupuncture can all potentially contribute to assisting with managing stress and anxiety (MHF, 2007:56).

Relaxation

One technique for promoting relaxation is the Benson method. Herbert Benson (1975) developed the technique for people with high blood pressure. He initially suggested that individuals sit still and quietly and focus on saying the word 'one' on their outward breath for a short duration of time, allowing the mind and body to slow down with no specific effort. The word 'one' can be replaced by other words that an individual may find more natural, such as calm, peace, love, still, silent, relax, ohm, etc.

The word, or mantra, can be spoken silently within rather than aloud and the technique can be used in everyday life, for example when queuing at a supermarket, on the train, while out walking, at an office desk, etc.

Adapted version of Benson method relaxation script

- Sit quietly with an open body posture.
- Focus on breathing.
- As you breathe out, focus on a desired word (for example, calm, one, peace, relax, joy).
- The word can be spoken aloud or quietly within.
- Practice this for about 5 minutes, just allowing the body to relax.

EXERCISE RECOMMENDATIONS

Stress may be the most common of the mental health conditions and it is certainly the one that most people report experiencing. With this in mind, it is recommended that you use the ACSM guidelines for the general population to prescribe a programme of exercise and activity. However, specific training recommendations for frequency, intensity, time and type should be considered in relation to each of the following:

- the existing fitness level and activity levels of the individual;
- the severity and longevity of their stress related condition;
- the individual's personal circumstances and support systems;
- the individual's previous and current medical history;
- the existence of other medical conditions that may be medicated; and
- the individual's current medications.

Exercise implications

The implications are specific to the condition, so know the client and their condition. General guidelines include:

- Advise clients with General Anxiety Disorder (GAD) or panic disorder of the initial effects of exercise (increased heart rate, etc.), so that symptoms are not mistaken for a panic or anxiety attack.
- Some clients with OCD may have to use their own equipment and will feel uncomfortable to share (contamination).
- Consider the risk of exercise becoming an obsession.
- Consider the side effects of medication.
- Create a positive environment using positive language and reinforcement.
- Teach relaxation techniques.
- Frequency, intensity, time and type should reflect individual needs.

- Deliver lower intensity versions first and offer progressions as an option.
- Promote a non-competitive atmosphere.

PSYCHOTIC CONDITIONS

These conditions are perhaps the most debilitating and enduring of the mental health conditions.

SCHIZOPHRENIA
Definition

The true definition of schizophrenia is 'disintegrative psychosis' from the Greek word for 'split mind', which is characterised by the splitting of normal links between perception, mood, thought, behaviour and contact with reality. It is definitely not the commonly perceived split personality.

Prevalence

It is estimated to affect 1 in every 100 people and the lifetime prevalence risk is 0.85 per cent. The peak age of onset is late adolescence/early adulthood and there are higher rates of diagnosis in African Caribbean and Black African men (DS-IV-TR, 2007).

Causes

As with most mental health conditions, there is no definitive cause, however there is a genetic link to a positive family history of the condition, with higher rates in identical twins than non-identical. Other suggested causes are neurodevelopmental or neurochemical damage, a history of cannabis use and social or environmental factors (DS-IV-TR, 2007).

Diagnosis

Schizophrenia is one of the most difficult disorders to categorise and diagnose as it can include the signs and symptoms of other categorised mental conditions. For example, the experience of extremes of elation or depression are characteristic of other disorders (bipolar – page 53, and depression – page 20).

Substance abuse may also cause symptoms that resemble schizophrenia (Spearing, 2009), and occasionally, people suffering with other undetected medical conditions experience severe mental symptoms and psychosis that resemble those of schizophrenia (Spearing, 2009). A comprehensive medical and physical examination is completed prior to diagnosis. A GP will ask about the symptoms being experienced, and will check that they are not the result of other causes, such as illegal drug use. Many people will fear diagnosis and the associated prejudice. However, early intervention is essential for a more successful treatment plan.

Diagnosis of schizophrenia may be based on the presence of first-rank symptoms (FRS) of schizophrenia, first described by Kurt Schneider in 1959. FRS includes certain types of auditory hallucination, namely a person discussing or making a running commentary about the patient, thought echo, withdrawal, insertion or broadcast. Other FRS include passivity (as state of being passive, submissive, inactive or acquiescent), somatic passivity (the delusion that an outside force is able to control bodily functions) and delusional perception (a delusion that arises in response to a normal perception).

Second-rank symptoms (SRS) include formal thought disorder and delusions. Symptoms are divided into **positive**, including hallucinations and delusions and **negative**, including poverty of speech, flat affect (lack of emotional response), poor motivation, social withdrawal and a lack of concern for social conventions. Symptoms can also be cognitive, including poor attention and memory.

The NHS (2010) suggests schizophrenia can usually be diagnosed if:

- at least two of the following symptoms are present:
  - delusions
  - hallucinations
  - disordered thoughts or behaviour
  - the presence of negative symptoms, such as a flattening of emotions;
- the symptoms have had a significant impact on the person's ability to work, study or perform daily tasks;
- the symptoms have been experienced for more than six months; and
- all other possible causes, such as recreational drug use or depression, have been ruled out.

If a GP suspects a diagnosis of schizophrenia, they may initially refer the person to a local community mental health team (CMHT), a group of mental health professionals who provide support to people with complex mental health conditions. A member of the CMHT team, usually a psychologist or psychiatrist, will carry out detailed assessment of symptoms, personal history and current circumstances and may use a diagnostic assessment (NHS, 2010).

Signs and symptoms

The symptoms used to define an acute episode are called positive symptoms and those that continue after the acute episode are referred to as negative symptoms (Davison & Neale, 2001).

Positive/acute symptoms

Hallucinations: One of the key symptoms of schizophrenia is hallucinations, which can be auditory (hearing things), visual (seeing things), olfactory (smelling things), gustatory (tasting things) or tactile (feeling things). Each of these can be very distressing and hard to shut out and often a person will have developed a coping strategy that helps them when hallucinations occur.

The most common of these is auditory hallucinations, commonly hearing voices. Using brain imaging techniques, researchers have shown that an area of the brain known as the Broca's area is active when voices are heard. This area is active when one has an internal conversation or speech – for example when rehearsing a presentation or speech – or when hearing voices. The difference between our 'normal' inner speech and hallucinations is that hallucinations also activate the auditory cortex of the brain, normally only activated when we are listening to exterior sounds such as music or someone talking as well resulting in a sensation of voice, which can be familiar or unfamiliar, coming from outside the brain.

The effect of hallucinations on a person's life can vary. For some the voices can be a comfort or an inspiration while for others they might be distressing or disturbing and can have a very negative effect, particularly if the voices are critical, hostile or demanding. In these cases, people can commit antisocial acts because of an 'order' from the voices. In some cultures, hearing voices is considered to be a gift and elevate the person to a higher rank.

Delusions: Spearing (2009) describes these as 'false beliefs that are not subject to reason or contradictory evidence and are not explained by the person's usual cultural concepts'. The NHS (2010) describes delusions as 'believing in things that are untrue'. Delusional symptoms can manifest in a patient as:

- feeling persecuted or conspired against by someone close to them.
- grandiosity, whereby the person believes they are a famous or important person believing that people on television are sending out messages specifically for them (Spearing, 1999; Davison & Neale, 2001).

Hallucinations and delusions are referred to as psychotic symptoms or psychosis. Psychosis occurs when the person is unable to distinguish between reality and their imagination.

Disordered thinking and speech: Thought patterns can be disorganised, fragmented and illogical. This can make conversation difficult, as there will be a tendency for sufferers to jump from one subject to another, which can contribute to social isolation.

Negative symptoms

Emotional expression: Persons with schizophrenia may display a 'flat affect', that is, they will not show the signs of normal emotion. They may speak in a monotone voice, sit for long periods without moving or making a sound, stare vacantly without facial expression, and can appear apathetic, with decreased motivation. They may also lose interest in daily routines (e.g. personal hygiene).

Other symptoms

Catatonia: This can include holding unusual positions for long periods, repeated gesturing of the upper limbs or waxy flexibility, whereby, the patient allows their body to become loose and will allow other people to move their body into unusual positions which they will then maintain (Davison & Neale, 2001).

Inappropriate affect: Emotional responses may be inappropriate for the context, for example, getting angry when asked a question or laughing at news of bereavement (Davison & Neale, 2001).

Prognosis

The NHS (2010) suggests that research has shown that out of 100 people with schizophrenia:

- 20 people will never have another acute schizophrenic episode;
- 50 people will experience a relapse of symptoms within 2 years;
- 30 people will never be free of symptoms, although the severity of symptoms can fluctuate over time; and
- 20 people will remain resistant to treatment and will require constant support and supervision.

The condition has a 10 per cent suicide rate and the prognosis is poorest in young males who are single, socially isolated, from a low social class, have misused drugs, show negative symptoms and have a family history of the condition.

Comorbidities

There are a number of physical conditions that are more prevalent in people with schizophrenia. Possibly due to the condition itself, the medications or the negative lifestyle behaviours commonly seen in schizophrenia, these need careful consideration when planning activity.

- Coronary heart disease occurs in 4 per cent of people with schizophrenia compared with 3 per cent of the general population and an increased mortality rate (1.1 times).
- 55 per cent are diagnosed under the age of 55, which compares unfavourably with the diagnosis rate of 18 per cent for the rest of the population.
- There are higher rates of hypertension and stroke and 21 per cent of strokes occur before the age of 55, almost double the rate in the rest of the population (11 per cent).
- Obesity rates are 33 per cent compared with 24 per cent of the general population, perhaps linked to a sedentary lifestyle but also a significant side effect of medications.
- Diabetes is diagnosed in 6 per cent compared with 2 per cent of the general population, possibly due to lifestyle factors but this can also be triggered by medication.
- There are higher rates of respiratory problems, perhaps not surprising given that over 70 per cent smoke compared with 23 per cent of the rest of the population, leading to a more than doubled rate of mortality. Again, the rate for diagnosis under 55 is significantly higher than for the general population at 23 per cent and 17 per cent respectively.
- There is also a link between schizophrenia and gastrointestinal problems, with nearly double the risk of premature death and a high incidence of bowel cancer.
- The risk of breast cancer is significantly higher in this group and due to the nature of the condition; these diseases may not be diagnosed early leading to a higher mortality rate.

- There are also higher rates of rheumatoid arthritis in people with schizophrenia.

The reasons for these higher risks are complex – possibly resulting from genetic factors, lifestyle and side effects of medications. The consequence is that people with severe mental illness are likely to die 10–15 years earlier than the remaining population and five-year survival rates for almost all these conditions are lower for people with mental health problems generally.

After five years, and adjusting for age:

- 22 per cent of people with coronary heart disease (CHD) who have schizophrenia have died, compared with 8 per cent of people with no serious mental health problems;
- 19 per cent of people with diabetes who have schizophrenia have died, compared with 9 per cent of people with no serious mental health problems;
- 28 per cent of people who have had a stroke and have schizophrenia have died, compared with 12 per cent of people with no serious mental health problems; and
- 28 per cent of people with chronic obstructive pulmonary disorder (COPD) who have schizophrenia have died, compared with 15 per cent of people with no serious mental health problems.

If nothing else, exercise and activity can at least reduce some of these risk factors for premature death.

Treatment

The first line of treatment for schizophrenia is usually a combination of antipsychotic medication, psychosocial interventions (e.g. CBT) and/or hospitalisation.

Medications work by increasing or reducing the effects of neurotransmitters such as dopamine, serotonin, noradrenalin and acetylcholine in the brain. These neurotransmitters regulate many aspects of behaviour including mood and emotions, control of sleeping, wakefulness and feeding.

Antipsychotic drugs

Antipsychotics are classified by their chemical structure and can be distinguished by their pharmacology (their action at different neurotransmitters receptors) and their clinical properties. The most commonly used system of classification refers to antipsychotics as either 'typical' or 'atypical' antipsychotics. The typical, or conventional, antipsychotics were first developed in the 1950s and act primarily to decrease the level of the neurotransmitter dopamine in the brain.

Atypical antipsychotics were first developed in the 1970s, followed by a new generation of atypical antipsychotics in the 1990s. Atypical antipsychotics are less likely than typical antipsychotics to cause movement disorders as a side effect, although they may still cause movement disorders when used at higher doses.

As with all medicines antipsychotics can produce side effects in some people. Some of the older medications have been shown to produce side effects that resemble the more difficult to treat symptoms (reduced motivation and emotional expression) and some can produce side effects that could aggravate other medical conditions. In addition, some people with schizophrenia can also become depressed and antidepressant medication can be added to their treatment plan. Adherence to medication is important because relapse may be more likely when medication is taken irregularly or discontinued. Spearing (2009) suggests that when a doctor says it is okay to stop taking a medication, it should be reduced gradually, never stopped suddenly.

The most common include movement disorders (referred to as extrapyramidal side effects) that may resemble Parkinson's Disease; dry mouth, blurred vision and constipation, feelings of dizziness or light headedness and weight gain. Rarely, antipsychotics may cause more serious side effects such as diabetes or metabolic syndrome, neuroleptic malignant syndrome (fever, faster breathing, sweating, muscle stiffness and reduced consciousness) and cardiac arrhythmias (irregular heart beat). They may also increase the risk of stroke in elderly people with dementia (by three times) and any patient who has pre-existing risk factors for stroke.

However, medications do not cure the condition, nor do they prevent the occurrence of future relapses into a psychotic episode, they control the symptoms of the condition. The majority of people show improvement when treated with antipsychotic medication.

Depot injections

Some antipsychotics are available as intramuscular (also known as 'depot' injection) usually into the hip, which can last in the system for between one and six weeks. This can help with compliance and reduce incidences of psychosis.

Electroconvulsive (ECT) therapy

The use of ECT is limited nowadays and is primarily used only in severe cases where all other treatment has failed. It is administered in hospital settings, and consists of passing a brief electrical current (between 1 and 4 seconds) through the brain with the use of anaesthesia and a muscle relaxant (Daines et al., 1997). It is used only with consent or if there is a risk to the client's life (Davison & Neale, 2001:264).

Other treatments

Psychological treatment is a broad term used to describe any therapeutic approach, which aims to adapt thought and behaviours, and it can be offered in conjunction with medication. These are some of the psychological treatments that may be on offer in different Health Boards:

Psychotherapy and counselling may not be a replacement for medication but can be very useful for supporting an individual through their experience and can help them explore and sort out the real from the distorted.

Cognitive behaviour therapy focuses on helping the person to manage the symptoms that do not go away even when they take medication. The therapist teaches the person how to check the reality of their thoughts and perceptions, how to 'not listen' to their voices, and how to manage their symptoms overall. CBT can help reduce the severity of symptoms and reduce the risk of relapse (Spearing, 2009). CBT is based on the theory that most unwanted thinking patterns and emotional and behavioural reactions are learned. The aim of CBT is for the person to:

* identify the thinking patterns that cause the unwanted feelings and behaviour; and
* learn to replace these with more realistic and helpful thoughts.

CBT is short-term intervention and usually requires between 8 and 20 one-hour sessions over the space of 6 to 12 months.

Group therapy can help those recovering from acute symptoms to explore some of their issues with others. It can provide a vital source of support for some people.

Family therapy explores the whole family as one unit in a time-limited, focused piece of intense work. Many people with schizophrenia rely heavily on other family members for care and support. The stress of caring for somebody with schizophrenia can place a strain on the family and family therapy offers a support mechanism. It involves a series of informal meetings over a period of six months and may include discussions about:

* information about the condition;
* ways of supporting the person; and
* finding solutions to practical problems that can be caused by the symptoms of the condition.

Rehabilitation or occupational therapy. Other non-medical interventions, such as life skills training, work and vocational training and counselling, social skills, and self-management skills are essential to assist the individual with re-integration into the community. Family education programmes can also assist other family members with supporting the individual and enabling them to cope more effectively. Many people with schizophrenia find that they benefit from meeting with an occupational therapist. Most CMHTs will have an occupational therapist working as part of the team. Occupational therapists can help to:

* identify both weaknesses and strengths;

* improve the patient's social and communication skills; and
* provide practical help and training for getting back to work.

Life in the community is becoming an important concept in improving the approach to mental illness. Key elements of this are enabling the person to take charge of his/her life with appropriate support and ensuring real choice for individuals (the person is 'empowered'). This is becoming more important as the emphasis is now on people living in the community, rather than spending a long time in hospital, so help may be needed to assist them to fulfil their potential. There are various forms of support aimed at helping someone regain confidence and self-esteem, and possibly building up everyday skills, including those needed to manage a household. Opportunities for daytime activity, including volunteering, are increasingly being made available.

Day care centres are organisations that provide services to assist and support persons with mental health conditions. They will deliver various life skills programmes that help the person to function healthily. Some of the services offered may include:

* programmes which support the development of ICT skills;
* financial advice and support;
* referral to exercise and activity programmes;
* cookery and healthy eating classes; and
* therapy.

Self-help/mutual support groups meet in many parts of the UK and include groups such as those run by the NSF (Scotland). Fife Hearing Voices Network can be a very useful complement or alternative to other forms of 'talking treatment'. They tend to be run, supported and used by individuals who are affected by hearing voices of some kind. There is good evidence that discussion among those who hear voices can help people to develop effective coping strategies. People with many different diagnoses (or none at all) find it helpful to get involved with Hearing Voices Groups.

Activity and diet: Attention to activity and diet is essential to reduce the risk of other medical conditions, such as heart disease, high blood pressure and diabetes.

Management

People with schizophrenia and other more complex mental health conditions, are usually entered into a treatment process, known as a 'care programme approach' (CPA). See appendix 3, page 178, for details.

Hospitalisation – voluntary or compulsory detention and advanced directives

This can be necessary for individuals who do not respond to medication or whose symptoms provide a potential risk for themselves (own health and safety, possible suicide) or safety of others. The Mental Health Act (1983 and 2007 – see appendix 5, page 181) informs procedures for hospitalisation and compulsory detention. People with schizophrenia will sometimes write an advanced directive that describes what they would like their family or friends to do in the event of an acute episode. This directive may include detention.

People with schizophrenia who are compulsorily detained may need to be kept in locked wards and will only stay as long as necessary for treatment. An independent panel will regularly review the case and progress. When they feel there is no risk to the person or others they will discharge them. However, the care team may recommend voluntary hospitalisation.

However, as Spearing (1999) reports, 'All too often, people with severe mental illnesses such as schizophrenia end up on the streets or in jails, where they rarely receive the kind of treatment they need'.

SCHIZOAFFECTIVE DISORDER
Definition
Schizoaffective disorder is a combination of mood and thinking problems so symptoms of mania or depression and psychotic symptoms of schizophrenia may be present at the same time or within days of each other (Rethink, 2010).

Prevalence
This disorder usually begins in late adolescence or early adulthood and there is a 1 in 200 (0.5 per cent) chance of developing schizoaffective disorder. It is more common in women than men (Rethink, 2010). However, some believe the low level of diagnosis does not represent the true prevalence and that many people are misdiagnosed. One clinical study showed that a quarter of all psychotic patients were eventually diagnosed with schizoaffective disorder (Rethink, 2010).

Causes
As with other psychotic disorders, the causes of schizoaffective disorder are unknown but it is thought that both genetic and environmental factors and chemical imbalances are contributory factors (see potential causes of schizophrenia,

pages 44–45) and stress may have a key role in triggering the condition.

Diagnosis

Diagnosis is distinguished from schizophrenia or bipolar disorder by the timing of symptoms. A schizoaffective episode must last for at least a month with mood problems and thinking disorders appearing simultaneously, however, the mood symptoms must disappear for at least two weeks during that time.

Signs and symptoms

Schizoaffective disorder shares the symptoms of both depression, bipolar and psychosis. Hypomania (mild to moderate mania) may feel good and may be associated with good functioning. Without proper treatment, hypomania can become either severe mania or depression may develop. One person may have more of one type of symptom than another, and may be diagnosed as having manic type, depressive type or mixed type schizoaffective disorder. It is possible to experience symptoms of one type during one episode, but have different symptom types during a different episode.

Manic type

Symptoms such as hallucinations or delusions may occur but are not necessarily either grandiose or paranoid. Manic type episodes usually start suddenly, with people behaving in a very disturbed way for a short time, making a full recovery within a few weeks. Manic type patients may be less vulnerable to relapse than depressive type.

Manic type symptoms

- Elation, increased self-esteem and unrealisable plans
- Excitement
- Irritability, with aggressive behaviour
- Increased energy
- Overactivity
- Inability to concentrate
- Uninhibited behaviour

Depressive type

Hallucinations or delusions can occur and are likely to be grandiose or paranoid. Depressive type is usually less dramatic and alarming than manic type, but is likely to last longer. Some schizophrenic symptoms may linger for a while.

Depressive type symptoms

- Feeling very low
- Feeling slowed down
- Insomnia
- No energy
- No appetite; losing weight
- Loss of usual interests
- Lack of concentration
- Feeling guilty
- Feeling hopeless
- Suicidal thoughts

Mixed type

Mixed type is diagnosed when symptoms of schizophrenia are co-existent with symptoms of bipolar disorder.

Treatment

A combination of drug treatments and psycho-social therapies will form part of the treatment plan, usually in conjunction with the community mental health team. Hospital care may be needed in more severe episodes. Medication will overcome the symptoms of psychosis while other therapies may be needed to overcome other associated problems (unemployment, homelessness, etc.).

Medication

As schizoaffective disorder combines symptoms of thought, mood and anxiety disorders, a combination of antipsychotic, antidepressant and anti-anxiety medications may be used.

- Antidepressants such as SSRIs may be prescribed for depressive type, however use is carefully monitored as they can trigger manic episodes.
- Antipsychotics may be prescribed in the short term to help with troublesome psychotic symptoms.
- Benzodiazepines may be used to reduce agitation and anxiety.
- Mood stabilisers such as lithium are used if mania or mood swings are present.
- ECT may also be used in very severe depressive or manic phases.
- If someone is not compliant with medication long-acting injections (depot) of antipsychotic medications are required.

Therapy

CBT is the preferred form of therapy for schizoaffective disorder as it is considered effective and group therapy is beneficial, particularly in an inpatient setting (Rethink, 2010).

Family therapy may help decrease relapse rates for those in high stress situations. In high-stress families, a person may have a 50–60 per cent relapse in the first year out of hospital. Supportive family intervention can reduce this relapse rate to below 10 per cent.

Behavioural therapy can successfully teach much needed social and occupational skills when psychosis has passed.

BIPOLAR DISORDER
Definition

Previously referred to as manic depression, bipolar disorder is an episodic condition characterised by periods of extreme highs (mania) and lows (depression) in a person's mood or emotions. It is described by some as like being on a rollercoaster, and can have a significantly debilitating effect on the lives of both the person and those around them. There are two main types of bipolar disorder, bipolar I and bipolar II.

Bipolar disorder is sometimes grouped with the psychotic disorders and sometimes with the mood disorders, as different variations of the condition share symptoms from both groups of conditions. During the high or manic phase delusions and hearing voices, which depict psychosis, may be experienced and during the low or depressed phase low mood and suicidal thoughts typical of major depression may occur.

Prevalence

Bipolar is considered a relatively common condition with around 1 person in 100 being diagnosed (NHS, 2010). Occurring at any age, it often develops between the ages of 18 and 24 years and can be triggered during times of physical and emotional stress, for example pregnancy and childbirth, menopause, during work, marital or family problems. Women are 1.5 times more likely to develop bipolar disorder than men and it affects people from all backgrounds.

Symptoms

Persons experiencing bipolar disorder may display a range of signs and symptoms ranging from extreme lows (during the depressive phase) to extreme highs (during the manic phase). The pattern of mood swings in bipolar disorder varies widely between individuals and according to the diagnosis. For example, some people will only have a couple of bipolar episodes in their lifetime, and will be stable in between, while others may experience many episodes and more severe symptoms.

The depression phase of bipolar disorder often comes first. Initially, the person may be diagnosed with clinical depression before experiencing a manic episode and receiving the diagnosis of bipolar, sometimes years later (Strock, 2000; Davison & Neale, 2001; NIMH, 2010).

Depressive phase

Some of the signs and symptoms include:

- sleep problems: insomnia (not sleeping) or hypersomnia (sleeping all the time);
- feelings of helplessness, worthlessness, guilt or hopelessness;
- inability to focus and/or concentrate;
- lethargy, apathy, low motivation and interest;
- eating disturbances, loss of appetite or rapid weight gain; and
- suicidal thinking or attempts.

Manic phase

Some of the signs and symptoms include:

- abnormal or excessive euphoria/elation;
- decreased need for sleep;
- high creativity;
- increased libido;
- grandiose notions;
- increased energy;
- irritability;
- rash and inappropriate social behaviour (e.g. overspending); and
- racing thoughts and speech.

Diagnosis

A GP will usually refer the person to a psychiatrist if they suspect bipolar disorder. If there is a risk of harm to the person or others, an immediate appointment will be arranged. A number of questions may be asked to confirm the diagnosis and identify the most appropriate treatments. Questions may include:

- the symptoms being experienced;
- when the symptoms started;
- feelings leading up to, and during, both the manic and depressive phases;
- the presence of any thoughts about harming self or others;
- medical background; and
- family history of bipolar.

Other tests may also be carried out, depending on the symptoms presented, for example, checks for other physical/medical problems such as thyroid disease.

Types of bipolar disorder

Bipolar I

This involves recurring phases or episodes of mania and depression (major or clinical depression) but is characterised mainly by a manic phase, followed by a period of depression. Some people with bipolar I may not experience the major or clinical depressive episode.

Bipolar II

This involves a longer lasting depressive phase alternating with phases of hypomania. The manic phase tends to be less disruptive and may not affect day-to-day functioning, as the symptoms of the manic phase are those considered less representative or psychotic in nature (e.g. increased energy or a more elated mood).

Cyclothymia

Cyclothymia is a less disabling and less severe variation and therefore does not warrant the full diagnosis. However, the symptoms will still prevent the person from feeling good about themselves and they may affect some functioning, but there is no drive to commit suicide. The symptoms need to be experienced for a longer period, approximately a period of two years before cyclothymia is diagnosed (Davison & Neale, 2001).

Rapid cycling bipolar

This involves rapid mood fluctuations between depression and hypomania or mania with very little or no period of stability (euthymia) between phases. It is diagnosed if four or more episodes that meet the criteria for the major depressive, manic, mixed or hypomanic phases occur during the course of a year. Some people experience monthly, weekly or even daily shifts between the mania and depression phases. The latter is sometimes called ultra rapid cycling (Rethink, 2010).

Mixed bipolar state

This involves symptoms of mania and depression occurring at the same time. The person may be experiencing a low mood but may also feel highly energised. Symptoms can include sleep problems, changes in appetite, feeling agitated, psychosis and suicidal thoughts (Rethink, 2010).

Causes

The exact cause is unknown, however, it is believed that a combination of social, physical and environmental factors may contribute to, and trigger, the condition.

Chemical imbalance

Bipolar disorder is believed to be the result of chemical imbalances in the brain. The chemicals or neurotransmitters that are responsible for controlling the functions of the brain include norepinephrine, serotonin, and dopamine. It is believed that an imbalance in the levels of one or more of these neurotransmitters may cause the symptoms of bipolar. For example:

- If norepinephrine levels are too high, this may cause a manic episode.
- If norepinephrine are too low, this may cause a depressive episode.

Genetic influences

Bipolar disorder is thought to have a significant genetic links, as there is evidence that it runs in families. Other family members of a person with the condition have an increased risk of developing bipolar (NHS, 2010). However, there is no single gene that is responsible, rather it is thought that a number of genetic and environmental factors act as 'triggers' for the condition.

Triggers

A stressful circumstance, or situation, is usually required to trigger the onset of the symptoms of bipolar disorder, but it may also be triggered by overwhelming problems in everyday life, such as struggles with money or at work and/or problems in relationships. Other examples of stressful triggers may include:

- Abuse: Physical, sexual, or emotional
- Relationship breakdown
- Bereavement: The death of a close relative, or loved one

These life-altering events can cause episodes of depression throughout a person's life. Struggling to cope with the symptoms of a physical or medical illness can also cause persistent periods of depression.

Prognosis

With regard to recovery, the prognosis following a manic episode is not good; nearly 90 per cent will experience a repeat episode, with an average of four episodes over a ten-year period. In bipolar I the frequency and severity of symptoms increases over the first four or five episodes and then plateaus. Those who show rapid cycling seldom respond to lithium and have a particularly poor prognosis. The course of cyclothymia tends to be chronic with nearly one-third developing bipolar disorder. Between episodes, with or without medication, people can experience long periods of euthymia, or stable emotions and live a relatively 'normal' life.

Comorbidity

Thirty per cent of people with bipolar disorder are clinically obese compared to 21 per cent of the rest of the population and the linked condition diabetes is more common in people with bipolar disorder (4 per cent) than the remaining population (2 per cent). Additionally, coronary heart disease is more common in people with bipolar disorder (5 per cent) compared with the rest of the population (3 per cent).

People with mental illness are also at higher risk of developing high blood pressure, stroke, respiratory problems and bowel and breast cancer. The reasons for these higher risks are not fully understood, but they may result from genetic factors, lifestyle and the side effects of medications. As a result, people with severe mental illness have a life expectancy 10–15 years lower than the remaining population. After five years, and adjusting for age:

- 15 per cent of people with bipolar disorder died, compared with 8 per cent of people with no serious mental health problems.
- 19 per cent of people with bipolar disorder had a stroke compared with 12 per cent of people with no serious mental health problems.
- 24 per cent of people with bipolar disorder had respiratory disease and chronic obstructive pulmonary disorder (COPD) compared with 15 per cent of people with no serious mental health problems.

Treatment

Someone with bipolar will need to visit their GP on a regular basis for other physical health checks. There may be other medical problems (comorbidities) and the side effects of prescribed medication may include weight gain, which will need to be managed.

Advanced directive

The person is always actively involved in their treatment plan. However, there may be times when they are unable to communicate their decisions. In these instances, an advanced directive will be obtained. An advanced directive is a set of written instructions provided by the person in advance and states what treatments and help they want, or do not want.

Medication

Bipolar disorder is usually treated with the mood-stabilising drug lithium, however, as this medication can take up to six weeks to take effect, antipsychotics are often used for rapid tran-quilisation in manic episodes. Lithium can reduce the frequency and severity of manic episodes so is particularly effective as a maintenance treatment. However, due to its effects on the liver, kidney and thyroid disturbance it needs careful monitoring. Additionally there is a risk of hypothyroidism which combined with the lethargic effect can lead to significant weight gain.

Anticonvulsants, including carbamazepine, sodium valproate and lamotrigine, are used in the treatment and management of bipolar disorder. Their main effect is to prevent relapses and help reduce rapid cycling.

Antidepressants are used to treat depressive phase, however, these may have a tendency to bring on a manic or rapid cycling episode so they are used in conjunction with a mood stabiliser to reduce this risk.

In addition to pharmacological treatment, patients are often given support in the form of therapy, not necessarily to treat the condition, but to help them come to terms with it and the effects it has on their behaviour and lifestyle.

Table 2.3	Antimanics/mood stabilisers/antidepressants used for bipolar disorder		
Generic name	**Used for**	**Action**	**Side effects**
Lithium	Extreme mood swings, manic depression, severe depression, self-harm	Frequency and intensity of mood swings	Muscle weakness, tremor, thirst/dry mouth, weight gain, nausea/vomiting, drowsiness, lethargy, blurred vision
Anticonvulsants: Carbamazepine, sodium valproate, lamotrigine	Prevention of relapse in mania or depression	May be used when lithium is not tolerated or effective	Drowsiness, dizziness, diplopia, decrease in coordination, oedema, agitation, rash, increased blood pressure
Antidepressants: SSRIs or tricyclics	May be used to treat depressive episodes	Decrease reuptake of serotonin	Nausea/vomiting, insomnia, drowsiness, anxiety, restlessness

Other treatments

Psychotherapy involves talking about feelings from the past and links to present behaviour patterns and developing strategies to overcome these feelings.

CBT examines the connections between thoughts and behaviour and identifies new thought patterns to enable cessation of previous negative behaviours and adoption of positive behaviours.

Social rhythm therapy is a type of behavioural therapy used to treat the disruption in circadian rhythms (circadian rhythms involve changes in our physical, mental and behavioural patterns occurring as a response to light and darkness and that follow a roughly 24 hour cycle) that are common in bipolar disorder. It follows a bio-psychosocial model and recognises that although the disorder is biologically, rather than emotionally, based, it cannot be fully treated with medication alone. It hypothesises that stressful events, disruptions in circadian rhythms and personal relationships, together with conflicts arising out of difficulty in social adjustment, often lead to relapses so addressing these factors can help with managing the condition.

Support groups are made up of people who have similar experiences and can be very helpful in reducing the feeling of isolation often brought on by mental health disorders.

Exercise can help with both the mental and physical consequences of bipolar disorder. It is widely documented that exercise has a beneficial effect on depressive mood states and the physical benefits help to reduce or remove the risk factors associated with inactivity and medication.

EXERCISE RECOMMENDATIONS

Schizophrenia, schizoaffective disorder and bipolar disorder are complex conditions and research continues to explore the causes, prevention and treatment of these illnesses. There is no evidence base from which to prescribe a specific exercise or activity intervention, as some people will be able to function 'normally' most of the time, and exercise may be part of their 'normal' daily life.

Table 2.4	Health activity guidelines (adapted from CMO, 'At least 5 a week', 2004)
Frequency	Work towards including activities into your daily routine on at least 5 days of the week.
Intensity	Working at a moderate level to feel mildly breathless, warm but comfortable (use the adapted RPE intensity scale provided in part 3, page 169, and aim to work between Level 3 and 4).
Time	Work towards performing the chosen activities for a total of 30 minutes (this can initially be broken down into 3 x 10 minute slots of activity or 2 x 15 minute slots of activity or 6 x 5 minute slots of activity), each day.
Type	Any activity that fits well into your daily lifestyle, for example, walking, active hobbies, structured exercise, sport activities or a combination of all of these.

NB: It is advisable that these guidelines be considered in relation to the individual client: The severity of their condition, their personal circumstances, previous medical history and any other medical conditions, and the setting within which their programme is managed.

Exercise professionals working with this population should conduct a detailed screening assessment and work with other health care professionals to identify ways of supporting the person. The specific diagnosis, severity of the condition, level of functioning, implications and side effects of specific medications and/or other treatments and existence of other medical conditions should be considered prior to making any exercise prescription or recommendations.

The DoH (1996) activity for health guidelines (see Table 2.4) is recommended as a starting point for assisting the maintenance of health and quality of life, as persons with mental health problems are prone to experiencing 'worse physical health than the rest of the population' (Halliwell, 2005:26).

Exercise implications

- Frequency, intensity, time, type of activity will be determined by other individual factors and by medication. Consider:
  - lower intensity;
  - shorter duration;
  - non-complex; and
  - accessible and engaging activities.
- Medication can have an effect on heart rate, blood pressure, energy levels and may contribute to weight gain. All of these must be accounted for prior to recommending any specific exercise programme.
- Comorbidities must be considered.
- The exercise professional would need additional training and support, so that they know how to recognise and manage a psychotic episode.
- The inclusion of specific moving relaxation techniques (e.g. tai chi) can be useful for persons who need to relax but are unable to lie or sit still.

- Involving the group in the set up of the room and equipment may appeal to some.

EATING DISORDERS
DEFINITION
The most important feature of eating behaviours classified by the ICD-10 and DSM-IV (anorexia nervosa, bulimia nervosa and binge eating disorder) is an intense fear of being overweight.

PREVALENCE
Eating disorders are more prevalent in white women living in industrialised countries, and more commonly from the middle/upper social classes, but are spreading to lower social classes (Davidson & Neale, 2001). They usually begin in the early to mid-teenage years after a period of dieting and the occurrence of a life experience that is stressful to the individual. This may include abuse (physical, mental, emotional or sexual).

They occur more often in people who have been overweight as children and the prevalence among boys and men is increasing. This may be because men are now seeking help for eating disorders rather than hiding them.

Eating disorders are also an issue for female athletes and are one of the key components of the female athlete triad of conditions (see Figure 2.4), each of which are viewed on a continuum of severity.

Bean (2010) evidences the following studies and findings:

- University of Leeds, UK (2001): 16 per cent of elite female, middle and long distance runners had anorexia or bulimia, compared with 1–2 per cent for the general population.

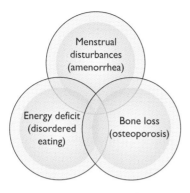

Figure 2.4 Female athlete triad

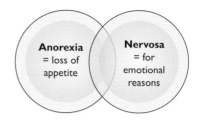

Figure 2.6 Definition of anorexia nervosa

- Norway (2004): 42 per cent of women competing at aesthetic sports and 24 per cent of women competing in endurance events met the clinical criteria for an eating disorder.
- University of Auburn, Montgomery, USA (1996): 23 per cent of female aerobics instructors had a history of bulimia and 17 per cent had a history of anorexia.
- Ball State University, USA (2002): 32 per cent of female athletes (sample size 425) had disordered eating, while 5.6 per cent were clinically diagnosed with an eating disorder.
- USA (2004): 30 per cent of female figure skaters considered themselves to be overweight and had a poor body image.

ANOREXIA NERVOSA
Definition

People suffering from anorexia do not actually lose their appetite or their interest in food. In fact, most are preoccupied with food and calorie counting. They have a distorted body image and an intense fear of gaining weight and will refuse to maintain a healthy body weight, normally weighing less than 85 per cent of their ideal body weight. This weight loss is primarily achieved by obsessive dieting, however excessive exercise, use of laxatives and vomiting may also be used. Someone with anorexia will monitor their weight gain and body measurements frequently and will critically evaluate their body image in a mirror. In some cases, menstruation may cease (amenorrhea).

Aesthetic sports	Endurance and low weight performance sports	Weight division sports	Gym sports
Gymnastics Ballet dance Synchronised swimming	Middle and long distance running Cycling Swimming Horse riding	Lightweight rowing Judo Karate Wrestling Boxing	Body building Aerobics Fitness

Figure 2.5 High-risk sports for eating disorders (Bean, 2010)

Prevalence

Anorexia typically begins during the teens and is 10 times more prevalent in females than men (Davison & Neale, 2001). The Royal College of Psychiatrists (2010) suggests that anorexia affects around:

- one fifteen-year-old girl in every 150; and
- one fifteen-year-old boy in every 1000.

It can also start in childhood or in later life. Anorexia has been linked with disturbances in the family environment or other life stresses apparent around this time. There may also be links with low levels of the neurotransmitter serotonin.

Signs and symptoms
Comorbidities and mortality

Key physical comorbidities in anorexia are gastrointestinal disorders, such as IBS, constipa-tion and bloating, osteoporosis due to the loss of menstruation, infertility and depression. Also common are reduced mobility and pain, dry skin, poor circulation leading to Raynaud's disease (also known as Raynaud's phenomon and which affects blood flow to the hands causing fingers to become cold and white, then blue then red, with sensations of numbness or pins and needles), perniosis (chillblains) and sleep disturbance.

Psychological comorbidities are depression, obsessive compulsive disorder (OCD), social phobia and avoidant personality traits. Mortality rates are higher amongst anorexics due to cardiovascular collapse, infections (including respiratory infections and tuberculosis (Morris, 2007)), and suicide, which has a higher incidence than any other psychiatric disorder and is 60 times that of the general population.

Table 2.5	Symptoms of anorexia nervosa	
Mental	**Physical**	**Behavioural**
• Can never be thin enough • Depression and anxiety associated with a distorted perception of body image and appearance • Intense fear of gaining weight • Self-esteem links to being thin	• Refusal to maintain a normal body weight • Excessive weight loss • Weigh less than 85 per cent of ideal body weight • Dull, thin and lifeless hair • Blotchy skin • Downy hair covering the body • Tiredness and lethargy • Poor healing of wounds • Sensitivity to cold • Loss of menstruation (amenorrhea)	• Obsessive dieting and calorie counting • Obsessive weighing and measuring of the body • Use of laxatives and excessive exercise to lose weight • Chew gum instead of eating • Mirror checking • In men or boys, erections and wet dreams stop, testicles shrink

Treatment

Talking therapies

A psychiatrist or psychologist will first want to talk with the person to find out when the problem started and how it developed. They will be weighed and may need a physical examination and blood tests (depending on weight loss). Family may also be consulted, with the permission of the person, however, this may not always be appropriate, especially in situations where abuse is suspected or where there are other family issues. All clients have the right to confidentiality, even the very young.

Therapy and counselling, where weight is checked and eating behaviours are monitored, provides the opportunity to explore issues that are upsetting and may be affecting eating behaviour (relationships, family problems, school, etc.). Therapy may be one to one or with small groups or other family members and can be ongoing for a number of years.

Hospital treatment

If the person is unable to maintain a healthy weight, they may be admitted to hospital. This also involves controlled eating and talking about problems in a more supervised and structured way. Some of the regular checks may consist of:

- Blood tests to check the risk of anaemia or infection.
- Weight checks to monitor weight gain.
- Other physical investigations to monitor any possible damage to other body systems (e.g. heart, lungs and bones).

How effective is the treatment?

More than half of sufferers recover, although on average, they may be ill for 5 to 6 years. Full recovery can happen even after 20 years of severe anorexia.

Past studies suggest that 1 in 5 of the most severely ill people admitted to hospital may die. However, the death rate is much lower, if the person stays in touch with up-to-date medical care. As long as the heart and other organs have not been damaged, most of the complications of starvation seem to improve slowly once a person is eating sufficiently (Rethink, 2010). 70 per cent of persons diagnosed with anorexia will recover, usually within 6 to 7 years.

BULIMIA NERVOSA

Definition

Bulimia is differentiated from anorexia because it is not associated with excessive weight loss. If weight loss is evident, anorexia is diagnosed.

The cycle of bulimia nervosa is dietary restriction followed by regular binges on excessive amounts of food (usually triggered by a negative emotion that the patient is unable to manage). This is then followed by purging behaviours (e.g. self-induced vomiting, use of laxatives and exercise) to prevent weight gain. The purging behaviours cause the individual to experience feelings of shame and remorse and contribute to maintenance of this destructive behaviour cycle.

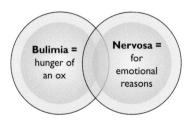

Figure 2.7 Definition of bulimia nervosa

Prevalence

Bulimia typically occurs in late adolescence and early adulthood. The individual is usually overweight before the onset of the disorder. About 4 out of every 100 women suffer from bulimia at some time in their lives, with fewer men, although the number of men affected is not currently known (Royal College of Psychiatrists, 2010).

However, people do not usually seek help for it until their early to mid-twenties because they are able to hide it, even though it affects their work and social life. People most often seek help when their life changes, for example during the start of a new relationship or having to live with other people for the first time (Royal College of Psychotherapists, 2010).

Signs and symptoms

See Table 2.6 for a breakdown of signs and symptoms of bulimia nervosa.

Prognosis

70 per cent of persons diagnosed will recover while 10 per cent will remain symptomatic.

Comorbidity and mortality

Physical comorbidities linked to bulimia include Russell's sign (callouses on hand), Mallory Weiss tears (oesophageal lacerations), dental erosion, facial purpura (purple discolouration of the skin) and conjunctival haemorrhage, which are the results of self-induced vomiting. Other gastrointestinal problems are linked to the use of laxatives.

Depression, personality disorders, anxiety disorders, substance abuse and conduct disorder exist comorbidly with bulimia. Bulimia is also associated with risk taking and self-harming behaviours such as stealing, illicit drug use and promiscuity (Davison & Neale, 2001).

Mortality is less common in bulimia than anorexia but is linked to suicide and cardiac arrhythmias.

Table 2.5	Symptoms of bulimia nervosa		
Mental	**Physical**	**Behavioural**	**Other**
• Depression and low self-esteem	• Same weight or weight gain • Lazy bowels due to laxative misuse and abuse • Damage to teeth caused by self-induced vomiting • Imbalance of natural body salts • Russell's sign (callouses on the hand)	• Secret behaviour cycle of purging and bingeing • Rapid consumption of large quantities of food (within 2 hours) followed by vomiting, fasting, excessive exercise	• Binges triggered by negative emotions • Feelings of shame and remorse attached to bingeing and vomiting • Callouses on knuckles

Treatment

Psychotherapy

Two kinds of psychotherapy have been shown to be effective in bulimia nervosa:

1 **CBT:** CBT looks at thoughts and feelings. The person will need to keep a diary of their eating habits to explore what triggers eating binges. Working with the support of a therapist, the person can then work out better ways of thinking about, and dealing with, these situations or feelings. The therapist will help the person to regain a sense of their own value as a person.

2 **Interpersonal therapy (IPT):** This focuses on the relationships the person has with other people. It helps the person to understand their relational and emotional needs and helps them to rebuild supportive relationships to serve these needs, rather than use eating.

Nutritional advice

A dietician will provide advice on healthy eating to help the person get back to regular eating and maintain a steady weight without starving or vomiting.

Medication

Antidepressants such as SSRIs can initially reduce the urge to binge, which can provide a support alongside other treatments (e.g. therapy) to kick-start recovery.

How effective is treatment?

There is evidence that a combination of medication and psychotherapy is more effective than either treatment on its own. Recovery usually takes place slowly over a few months or many years. About 50 per cent of bulimics recover partially, cutting their bingeing and purging by at least half. This outcome is lower for persons using drugs and/or alcohol or for those who are self-harming.

BINGE EATING DISORDER (BED)

Formerly known as 'non-purging bulimia', this condition involves binge eating but without the purging of bulimia. Individuals with BED are likely to be overweight or obese but still have the desire to restrain or control their eating patterns in order to lose weight while conversely desiring to stabilise eating patterns and regain control of their lives.

BED has a higher prevalence than the other eating disorders classified. It is differentiated from anorexia because there is no weight loss and it can be differentiated from bulimia because there are no compensatory behaviours (e.g. purging, excessive exercise) that follow the bingeing. It is closely associated with obesity and a history of dieting. It also has links with depression, substance abuse and low self-esteem. Other contributory risk factors may include childhood obesity,

Bingeing

- Raiding the fridge
- Buying lots of fattening foods that you normally would not eat and eating it all in secret
- Eating lots of food in a short time span (a couple of hours), e.g. packets of biscuits, several boxes of chocolates and a number of cakes
- Taking other people's food
- Shoplifting to satisfy binge urges

constantly hearing critical comments regarding body weight and appearance (through teasing and bullying), low self-concept, depression and physical and sexual abuse.

Eating disorders not otherwise specified (EDNOS)

The diagnosis of EDNOS may be given to someone who is suffering from disordered eating (e.g. calorie counting, bingeing, purging etc.), but does not show all the symptoms described by the 'text book' definition of anorexia nervosa or bulimia nervosa. For example, the person may meet all the criteria for anorexia nervosa but may still have regular menstruation or despite substantial weight loss, their current weight is still within the normal range.

Other eating disorders include those where the person eats items not usually eaten, such as paper or dog biscuits.

The National College of Psychiatrists provide helpful fact sheets for person with anorexia and bulimia and binge eating disorder (see references, page 192).

Case study

Pauline, aged 46 always had confidence issues when she was younger. 'I thought I was fat and ugly. Now I am in my forties and I look at photographs of myself, I realise that I never valued myself or how beautiful I really was. I would binge eat and then purge by making myself sick or taking laxatives. I remember have a binge urge one day and there was nothing in the house to eat, so I ate a packet of dog biscuits! It was part of the whole self-loathing issue I was going through.'

BODY DYSMORPHIC DISORDER (BDD)/BODY IMAGE DISTURBANCE (BID)

BDD and BID are known precursors for eating disorders in those at risk. Body image is a complex combination of factors and while it is estimated that, for example, 50 per cent of American women are dieting, few have realistic expectations of an achievable body image. It is estimated that while over 80 per cent of women report being dissatisfied with their body image, many are not seeing an accurate reflection (Fox, 1997), and that for a minority more serious conditions develop such as depression.

Disordered eating and yo-yo or extreme dieting are often seen as a way of solving 'problems'

Case study

At 18, Kathryn, aged 31 became very weight conscious and started dieting to lose weight. 'I became obsessed with diet magazines and calorie counting and ate virtually nothing. I would sometimes go for a run, with my body wrapped in plastic bags. My weight dropped from 10.5 stone to 8.2 stone and my periods stopped. I was not diagnosed with an eating disorder, but my eating behaviour was disordered, in that I would deliberately eat very little.

On reflection, it was good to be in control. This was the only thing in my life I felt in control of at that time. My father was quite controlling and there was lots of other stuff going on in my life and I had not made the transition to independence.

I was one of the lucky ones – I think it was a phase I went through … some people are not that lucky.'

and improving body image, however, research suggests that for nearly one-quarter of dieters it can lead to anorexia or bulimia and both BDD and BID are diagnostic criteria for these conditions (Hawkins, 2009). However, for a minority, this distortion of body image can lead to more serious and drastic attempts to achieve a (usually unrealistic) ideal shape.

Causes

Numerous theorists put forward arguments as to what causes disordered eating behaviour.

Biological vulnerability

Studies by biological theorists indicate that there may be a genetic predisposition that contributes to the development of disordered eating behaviour. However, although there is confirmation that eating disorders run in families and that genetic transmission is a possible link, the precise mechanism is not yet known (Morris, 2007).

Psychosocial vulnerability

It is suggested that eating disorders share characteristics with other mental health conditions that may be risk factors. Precursors to an eating disorder are stress, unhappiness and low self-esteem. Abuse and hardship also feature in the lives of individuals with an eating disorder. These issues become mixed with thoughts about shape and weight and eating patterns that are out of proportion with 'normal' weight issues.

Hunger recognition

Most people know when they are hungry and need to eat. People with anorexia may not have this same recognition and can go without food to keep their body weight dangerously low.

Psychodynamic

Psychodynamic theorists suggest that disturbances between parent and child relationships are a contributory factor to disordered eating.

Systemic theories

Systemic theorists indicate that when a family presents a child with an eating disorder, it may be a way for the family to avoid other conflicts within the family (distraction). It may also be a way for the individual to have some control over their life within a disturbed or dysfunctional family system. Alternatively, eating is an important part of family life. Accepting food gives pleasure and refusing it will often upset someone. Saying 'no' to food may be the only way some people can express their feelings, or have any say in family matters.

Anorexia can also offer a sense of control. It can be very satisfying to diet as there is a feeling of achievement when the scales indicate that a couple of pounds have been lost. It is good to feel control over ourselves in a clear, visible way and for some this may be the only part of their life over which they feel they have control. This can become addictive.

Anorexia can also be an attempt to stop the transition to adulthood as it reverses some of the physical changes, including getting pubic and facial hair in men, breasts and menstrual periods in women. It is thought that persons with anorexia may be trying to delay the demands of getting older, particularly those related to sex.

Critical life events and emotional distress

Anorexia and bulimia can be related to numerous stressful life events, such as:

- physical illness;
- bereavement – loss of a loved one;

- the break-up of a relationship;
- marriage or leaving home;
- general life difficulties; and/or
- sexual or other abuse.

However, for some the eating disorder can continue when the original stress has passed. They may continue to feel uncomfortable or be fearful of eating or use the disorder as a form of control.

Depression/comfort eating

Many people with bulimia are often depressed, and initially, binge eating is a way of coping with feelings. However, after bingeing, guilt or self-disgust occurs so vomiting and laxatives are used to compensate for the eating behaviour, which can leave them feeling worse.

Cognitive theorists

Cognitive theorists identify personality traits, such as perfectionism and low self-esteem being common among persons with eating disorders. People with anorexia and bulimia often think less favourably of themselves and losing weight can be a way of trying to regain a sense of respect and self-worth.

Socio-cultural theories

Numerous socio-cultural factors have the potential to contribute to disordered eating. These include:

- society's obsession with the ideal body image;
- specific cultural standards and ideals established for the ideal body image;
- the influence of the media;
- the influence of the diet and exercise industry;'
- the individual perception of body image; and/or
- cultural attitudes, beliefs and perceptions.

Societies that do not value thinness have fewer eating disorders. Places where thinness is valued, such as ballet schools, bodybuilding gyms, gymnastic schools and some athletic and swimming clubs have more eating disorders (both in women and men). In western culture 'thin is beautiful' and the media promotes this image (see Figure 2.8). Television, newspapers and magazines show pictures of idealised, artificially slim people.

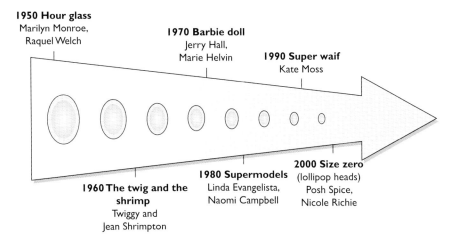

Figure 2.8 Changing standards representing the 'ideal' body image in western society

Interestingly, Davison & Neale (2001) reveal that to achieve the 'Barbie doll' ideal the average woman would need to:

- increase her bust size by 12 inches;
- reduce her waist size by 10 inches; and
- grow in height to over 7 feet.

Other cross-cultural considerations that may influence body image include:

- women being valued for their appearance;
- men being valued for their accomplishments;
- dancers and gymnasts and other female athletes needing to maintain a low weight to participate in their chosen activity (see the female athlete triad, Figure 2.4, page 59);
- industrialisation, which is eating disorders more common in industrialised countries; and
- cultural perceptions. One cross-cultural study revealed that Ugandan students rated obese women as more attractive than emaciated women whereas British students rated emaciated women as more attractive (Davison & Neale, 2001).

Comorbidities

Eating disorders are associated with a range of other mental health conditions including depression, personality disorders, anxiety disorders and substance abuse (addictions). They are also linked to self-harm and suicide. The disordered eating and exercise behaviours that accompany each disorder will also contribute to the longer term onset of other medical conditions, such as osteoporosis, obesity and congestive heart failure.

Treatment

Numerous interventions are suggested as part of the treatment plan for eating disorders. Those selected will be determined by the specific eating disorder.

Hospitalisation

If weight loss is excessive and there is a need for feeding, or if there is high risk of self-harming, the patient may be hospitalised.

Dietary advice

Re-education of eating perceptions through appropriate advice and support may assist with the return of functional behaviours and a healthy self-perception.

Talking therapies

Counselling and therapy (individual and group): Counselling and therapy can help the individual develop a healthy self-image and manage negative feelings. It may also help the individual to develop a greater insight into the causes of their behaviour, which in turn, can help them to manage specific events (e.g. stress or family patterns).

CBT: Cognitive and behavioural therapy focuses on thinking and behaviour.

Psycho-dynamic therapy: This focuses on the parent-child relationships and the links to self-esteem and perfectionism.

Family therapy: This involves treating the whole family and exploring family conflicts that the condition may be a distraction from (e.g. neglect, abuse, etc.).

Group therapy with other persons recovering from eating disorders can remove feelings of isolation and recognise shared experiences.

Medication

In some instances, medication may be prescribed as an intervention. Antidepressants may be prescribed to treat depressive symptoms. Additionally, other medication may be prescribed to stimulate appetite.

Exercise recommendations

There is no specific evidence-based guidance for working with persons with eating disorders. A key issue for consideration is that some clients with some eating disorders will be using exercise as a way of controlling their weight and may be at risk of over-exercising. This may include those from high-performing and endurance sports.

The Activity for Health guidelines and ACSM guidelines offer healthy and safe preliminary targets for both physical activity and physical fitness. Recommendations include:

- reviewing current activity and exercise levels to find a starting point for the person;
- encouraging safe levels of activity and exercise, within specific guidance frames;
- identifying different types of exercise to ensure that one specific mode is not over-used (encourage cross training, swimming, walking, gym-based, stretching, etc.);
- encouraging specific techniques that promote positive self-talk. Affirmations are also useful to assist with the development of a positive attitude, which can carry over into other areas of the person's life;
- valuing the person and supporting them, without colluding with unhealthy behaviours; and
- collaborating with other professionals working with the individual.

DISORDERS DUE TO PSYCHOACTIVE SUBSTANCE MISUSE

Substance misuse can be classified as either dependence or misuse. Dependence is considered the most serious because it involves a physiological addiction and physical dependence on the drug/substance used, i.e. the person experiences withdrawal symptoms when they are not using the drug and may have a high tolerance level (a need for more of the drug to get the same effects).

DEFINITION

The Diagnostic and Statistical Manual of Mental Disorders (DSM-IV-TR, 2000) defines substance misuse as:

a) A maladaptive pattern of substance use leading to clinically significant impairment or distress, as manifested by one (or more) of the following, occurring within a 12-month period:

- Recurrent substance use resulting in a failure to fulfil major role obligations at work, school, or home (e.g. repeated absences or poor work performance related to substance use; substance-related absences, suspensions or expulsions from school; neglect of children or household)
- Recurrent substance use in situations in which it is physically hazardous (e.g. driving an automobile or operating a machine when impaired by substance use)
- Recurrent substance-related legal problems (e.g. arrests for substance-related disorderly conduct)
- Continued substance use despite having persistent or recurrent social or interpersonal

problems caused or exacerbated by the effects of the substance (e.g. arguments with spouse about consequences of intoxication, physical fights)

b) The symptoms have never met the criteria for substance dependence for this class of substance. Substance dependence or addiction is diagnosed by DSM-IV if at least three of the following are presented:

- Tolerance, either by needing additional doses to provide the same effect or the effects of the drug becoming markedly less, with the same dosage
- Withdrawal – negative symptoms experienced when the drug is not used
- Withdrawal from other past times to use the drug (work, recreation and social)
- Using the drug more often and for longer
- The person recognises their over-usage but cannot stop
- A lot of time is taken to access the drug or recover from its effects
- The drug is taken despite physical or psychological problems being experienced (e.g. smoking and drinking and being aware of the health risks)

Broadly, the term 'misuse', used interchangeably with 'abuse', refers to the improper, illegal or harmful use of any substance, both legal and illicit. It is often linked with addiction, a compulsive physiological and/or psychological need for a habit-forming substance. The two main types of drug addiction are:

1 physical addiction, which leads to withdrawal symptoms, such as nausea, vomiting or cramping, if the drug is suddenly withdrawn and

2 psychological addiction, which involves a psychological compulsion or need to use a drug, with psychological symptoms such as depression and anxiety, occurring if the drug is withdrawn. There may be no physical withdrawal symptoms in psychological addiction.

Figures from the Home Office show that in the UK around 1 in 10 people have used illegal drugs in the last year, and 1 in 20 have used illegal drugs in the last month. It is important to note that because a drug is legal, it does not mean it is harmless. The legal drugs, cigarettes and alcohol, kill more people in England and Wales each year than all illegal drugs put together and prescription medications, such as strong painkillers or tranquilisers, are often misused by people who have no clinical need for the drug but use it for its mood-altering effects.

The many substances that are misused fall broadly into five categories:

1 Alcohol
2 Illicit or 'street' drugs
3 Prescription and over-the-counter medicines
4 Volatile substances
5 Nicotine, caffeine, colas and the rest

ALCOHOL MISUSE
Definition
Alcohol misuse is characterised by regular, heavy or binge consumption of alcohol in quantities sufficient to cause physical, neuropsychiatric or social damage.

Background

Perhaps one of the most 'accepted' forms of substance misuse relates to alcohol – it is legal, it is a normal part of everyday life for many and it is easily available. Approximately 90 per cent of the population consumes alcohol and the majority enjoy alcohol within safe limits (3–4 units per day for men and 2–3 units for women) with at least two alcohol-free days per week. Unfortunately, for many people alcohol contributes to physical and mental health problems despite its acceptable role as a positive and enjoyable part of life, and as an aid to stress management.

More than 800,000 people per year (1,000 under the age of 14) are admitted to hospital with alcohol-related injuries and illness, 6 per cent of all NHS admissions are in some way drink related and an estimated £25 billion annual bill for alcohol abuse falls on the taxpayer making it a major health issue. It is estimated that 40 per cent of men and 30 per cent of women regularly exceed the safe guidelines (see above).

Every year more than 4,000 people die from liver cirrhosis and around 700 need a liver transplant in the UK. There has been a 17.2 per cent increase in alcoholic-related liver disease, over the last 15 years. Figures for Scotland are worrying as the mortality rate in Scotland is the highest in the UK, with the percentage of men and women dying from alcohol-related illnesses more than double that in England and Wales. In 2001 Scotland had rates of 34 alcohol-related deaths per 100,000 for men and 16 for women. This compares to 14 for men and 7 for women in England and Wales (NTS, 2009).

Table 2.7	Change in annual pure alcohol intake in litres and source drink				
Year	Beer	Spirits	Wine	Cider	Total
1957	3.88	0.82	0.31	0.11	5.12
2007	4.48	2.40	3.52	0.81	11.2

Table 2.8	Disorders associated with alcohol misuse
Disorder	Symptoms
Acute intoxication	Slurred speech, impaired coordination or judgement
Acute withdrawal (occurring within 24–48 hours of abstinence)	Malaise, nausea, autonomic hyperactivity, insomnia, hallucinations/illusions
Alcohol dependence	Compulsion to drink, preoccupation with alcohol, altered tolerance of intoxicant effects
Psychotic disorders	Alcoholic hallucinosis, pathological or morbid jealousy

Prevalence/epidemiology

Harmful drinking is the consumption of more than 50 units for men and 35 units for women per week – an average of 7 units and 5 units per day respectively. To put it into perspective, that is the equivalent of two pints of strong beer or two glasses of 14 per cent wine. A total of 8 per cent of men and 2 per cent of women currently drink at these levels and the figures for women and adolescents are increasing. A binge is classified as drinking more than twice the daily limits in one session.

Diagnosis

Diagnosing alcohol misuse or addiction is not easy, as many people do not seek medical help or advice in early stages. Identification of 'at risk' individuals and thorough screening may help to prevent problem drinking becoming an addiction.

Diagnosis of alcohol dependence or addiction is made using an interview and discussing the 'typical drinking week', and there are two key questionnaires used to gain information about alcohol problems, FAST and CAGE (Semple et al., 2005).

Frequency of Alcohol Scoring Test (FAST)
Score the frequency of:

- more than eight drinks (men)/six drinks (women) on more than one occasion;
- the inability to remember the night before;
- the failure of normal functioning due to alcohol; and
- any relative/friend/health professional concerned about a person's drinking.

Answers: Never = 0. Continue beyond Q1 only if score is more than 0.

Q 1–3. Less than once a monthly = 1, monthly = 2, weekly = 3, daily = 4
Q4. No = 0, once = 2, more than once = 4
If the total score is greater than 2 it indicates hazardous drinking.

CAGE questions
Cut down: Have you tried to cut down?
Annoyed: Have people annoyed you by suggesting you do so?
Guilty: Have you felt guilty about drinking?
Eye-opener: Have you needed a drink first thing in the morning as an eye-opener?

Once an alcohol-related problem has been diagnosed there are many further assessments that are done to determine the extent of the problem, the likely cause, effects and appropriate treatment prescription.

Causes

What causes alcohol misuse or dependence? It is difficult to give a definite cause as there are many variants that can be considered influencing factors. However, there are distinct patterns that are seen in excessive alcohol consumption that warrant discussion.

Genetic factors/ethnicity
Alcohol dependence and misuse is high in Native Americans and Australians but low in Chinese and Japanese people.

Other genetic factors include the production of higher quantities of acetaldehyde that causes a flush reaction and significantly greater 'hangover' effect due to a genetic mutation in the acetaldehyde deydrogenase-2 gene. This occurs in approximately 50 per cent of Japanese individuals.

Heredity and a family history of depression are also linked to alcohol misuse.

Social factors

Occupation is a significant factor; alcohol misuse is higher in publican and bar staff and the armed forces (seafaring) (ONS, 2007).

Culture/peer group influences play a part – alcohol use is already low in those of Jewish or Muslim faith where alcohol and drunkenness are against beliefs, and it is higher in those of Scottish or Irish nationality.

Imitation and vicarious learning (unconscious learning via observing others) are also linked to misuse. Growing up in an environment where alcohol is misused predisposes to developing a problem. Social reinforcement is both a cause and disguise as the association between drinking and social occasions not only encourages the consumption of alcohol but can also mask overconsumption if everyone is drinking at the same (or perceived same) pace.

Cost

Cost of alcohol is also a factor; misuse is more prevalent in countries where it can be obtained cheaply and easily. In the UK a two-litre bottle of strong cider costs relatively little compared to a half bottle of whisky, yet contains more units of alcohol and is more palatable to adolescents.

Other factors

Alcohol is also used as a coping strategy by many: 'I need/deserve a drink, the sun is over the yard arm, finished work, kids are in bed' thinking can lead to habitual drinking and/or drinking in the day to avoid withdrawal symptoms.

Levels of alcohol consumption are higher in those with a chronic physical illness, particularly if there are high levels of pain, and in psychiatric illness such as mood and anxiety disorders.

Effects of alcohol misuse

There are many problems associated with alcohol misuse and the higher the consumption the greater risk of these. Individuals who drink within recommended limits are unlikely to experience harmful effects and there may be cardio-protective benefits from drinking within the limits for women post-menopause and men over 45.

Cardiovascular system

Problems associated with the cardiovascular system include coronary heart disease and cardiovascular disease, including peripheral arterial disease, anaemia and heart failure. The risk of stroke, hypertension and arrhythmias also increases if the limits are exceeded regularly.

Gastrointestinal and digestive systems

Regular or excessive use of alcohol can lead to stomach ulcers particularly if medicines containing aspirin are taken to relieve hangovers. Lack of or malabsorption of nutrients can lead to health problems, particularly if food is avoided to keep calorie counts down.

Pancreatitis is another result of excessive alcohol consumption and can lead to type II diabetes. Alcohol lowers blood glucose levels thereby increasing the risk of hypoglycaemia in individuals already diagnosed with diabetes. Furthermore, liver disease and cancer are linked with alcohol intake. There is also an increased risk of stomach, rectal and bowel cancer.

Neurological systems

The nervous system is also affected, with up to 25 per cent of alcohol dependents experiencing peripheral and autonomic neuropathy leading to numbness, gangrene and cerebellar degeneration or brain shrinkage leading to dementia.

Two neurological conditions caused by alcohol misuse are Wernicke's encephalopathy, which is the result of thiamine deficiency and causes acute confusion and ataxia, nystagmus (an uncontrolled and usually sideways movement of the eyes) and opthalmoplegia (weakness or paralysis of eye muscles). This can then develop into the more severe Korsakoff's psychosis/syndrome which is characterised by profound short-term memory loss and confabulation – giving fictitious accounts of past events, while believing they are true, to cover gaps in memory.

Other effects

Further health problems include gout, and cancer of the mouth, pharynx and larynx, oesophagus and breast. Reduced fertility levels, impotence and shrunken genitals are all effects of alcohol misuse. Drinking while pregnant, particularly in the early stages, can lead to foetal alcohol syndrome as alcohol crosses the placental barrier and can affect growth of the foetus, which can lead to facial stigmata, brain and neurological damage and cause psychological, behavioural and developmental problems, including learning disability, in the child.

Approximately 40 per cent of people attending Accident and Emergency departments have alcohol-related injuries or illness and its use is implicated in fires, domestic accidents, drowning, hypothermia and suicide.

Social effects

The deterioration in well-being and performance has consequences for other areas of life. There are increased marital problems and domestic violence associated with alcohol misuse, and poor performance at work can lead to unemployment or redundancy. Criminal activity such as shoplifting, theft, prostitution and driving offences are increased among this group. With regard to driving offenses, driving while over the legal limit makes you 10 times more likely to have an accident and 40 per cent of pedestrians killed in road traffic accidents had alcohol levels over the driving limit.

Prognosis

The prognosis for those with an established problem is mixed. One-third will have a positive outcome, that is abstinence or control of alcohol that results in a relatively normal life. Unfortunately, for the remaining two-thirds the outlook is not good. Alcohol misuse results in lifelong problems for approximately 30 per cent of the remainder, and for over half the sad effect is either premature death (40 per cent) or suicide (15 per cent).

Treatment

Motivational interviewing

This technique aims to help a client to move through the stages of change and into action. Discovering the cause of the problem and finding motivation to overcome it are key in recovery. As with smoking cessation, a person needs to want to change their behaviour in order to have a reasonable chance of success. Motivational interviewing is a guiding process led by the client and encourages client responsibility for both the problem and recovery.

Abstinence

Acute detoxification involves abstaining from alcohol for a period to allow the body and liver to detoxify and start to heal. This can be a very difficult process and may be done in a residential setting to aid recovery. There will need to be a support system in place once the patient is back in the community to prevent relapse.

Controlled drinking

Some clients may prefer to choose controlled drinking or a safer drinking pattern rather than abstinence and this may be successful if there is a history of success using this route in the past or if the drinking was part of a psychiatric problem that has been treated successfully. The social environment is also important as there needs to be an absence of alcohol-related problems in family and friends.

Therapy

The use of various forms of therapy, discussed fully elsewhere in this book, can also help to identify the root problems that may have led to alcohol misuse. The therapy must be chosen to suit the client to have the greatest chance of success.

Self-help groups (AA)

Groups like Alcoholics Anonymous (AA) can be effective in coping with an alcohol-related problem and for those who need support from other victims it is a positive route to changing behaviour.

Medication

Disulfiram is an aversive drug – it works by inhibiting acetaldehyde dehydrogenase, which converts alcohol to water and carbon dioxide. If alcohol is consumed, there is a build up of acetaldehyde in the system and this causes a range of unpleasant symptoms such as flushing, nausea, vomiting, tachycardia and headache. Acamprosate and naltrexone are anti-craving drugs. Both drugs have an effect on alcohol cravings, acamprosate reduces cravings and naltrexone reduces the 'high' that in turn reduces the desire for alcohol. Benzodiazepines are also used to control or minimise withdrawal symptoms.

Activity

Physical activity and exercise can be an aid to recovery as it helps to fill the gap created by disuse of alcohol and distract from withdrawal symptoms and stress, creating a positive behaviour habit. It also benefits physical health and can help to improve self-esteem and self-efficacy (a person's belief in their capabilities of achieving a goal) and create a sense of 'health' that has been lacking.

One study into residential treatment of alcoholics found that 69 per cent of those whose treatment included a daily programme of vigorous activity remained sober at a three-month follow up while 62 per cent who had not received the activity intervention had relapsed. Furthermore, a scheme in Scotland found that participants in activity reported benefits that included 'having something to look forward to – something that made you feel good'. Exercise and activity are discussed in further detail in chapter 3 (see page 84).

SUBSTANCE MISUSE

Socially less acceptable than alcohol abuse and seen as something of an antisocial and underclass problem, this is a worrying trend in the UK, particularly with the rise of so-called 'legal' highs.

Definition

Substance misuse is characterised as regular or excessive use of a substance that causes psychological, physical or social problems.

Dependence

Physiological dependence includes a withdrawal state or tolerance and involves a sense of compulsion to take the substance, difficulty in controlling use, increasing time spent obtaining, ingesting or recovering from the substance, persistence with substance use despite awareness of harmful consequences and a persistent but futile wish to cut down use. Other effects are the reduction or neglect of important social, occupational or recreational activity due to

Table 2.9 Substance misuse	
Use	**Resulting in**
Acute intoxication	Transient disturbances of consciousness, cognition, perception, affect or behaviour following administration of a psychoactive substance.
At-risk use	A pattern of use where an individual is at increased risk of harm to their physical or mental health.
Harmful use	Damage to the individual's health and adverse effects on family and society.

Table 2.10 Disorders associated with substance misuse	
Disorder	**Symptoms**
Withdrawal state	Physical and psychological symptoms occurring on absolute or relative withdrawal of a substance after repeated and prolonged and/or high dose use. Onset and course of withdrawal state are time limited and depend on type of substance and dose used.
Psychotic disorder	Psychotic symptoms occurring during or immediately after substance use, vivid hallucinations, abnormal affect, psychomotor disturbances, persecutory disturbances and delusions of reference.
Amnesic disorder	Memory and other cognitive impairments caused by substance use.
Residual and late onset psychotic disorders	Effects on behaviour, affect, personality or cognition lasting beyond the period during which a substance effect may be expected, e.g. LSD flashbacks, alcoholic hallucinosis, drug-induced psychosis.

Source: DSM-IV-TR, 2000 and Craig & Davies, 2009

substance use. Substance dependence or addiction is diagnosed by DSM-IV if at least three of the following are presented:

- Tolerance, either by needing additional doses to provide the same effect or the effects of the drug becoming markedly less, with the same dosage
- Withdrawal: Negative symptoms being experienced when the drug is not used
- Withdrawal from other past times to use the drug (work, recreation and social)
- Using the drug more often and for longer
- The person recognises their over usage but cannot stop
- A lot of time is taken to access the drug or recover from its effects
- The drug is taken despite physical or psychological problems being experienced (e.g. smoking and drinking and knowing the health risks)

Background

There are a wide range of drugs and substances that are misused and sadly more are becoming available. In particular, the so-called 'legal highs' include substances that can be legally obtained – though often they are not designed for or tested for human consumption, making them particularly dangerous.

Prevalence

It is difficult to monitor the use of illicit substances for obvious reasons but data from the NHS Treatment Agency (2009) and British Crime Survey (2006/7) collated from people seeking treatment shows the following estimates of drug use in England and Wales. Additional figures show that

Table 2.11	Drugs used in 2009 by 16–59 year olds		
Class	**Drug**	**Estimated no. of users**	**Percentage of population**
Class A	Cocaine	828,000	2.6
	Crack cocaine*	58,000	0.2
	Ecstasy	567,000	1.8
	Heroin*	41,000	0.1
	LSD	77,000	0.2
	Magic mushrooms	201,000	0.6
Class A/B	Amphetamines	421,000	1.3
Class B/C	Tranquilisers	136,000	0.4
Class C	Anabolic steroids	32,000	0.1
	Cannabis	2,616,000	8.2
Not classified	Amyl nitrate	440,000	1.4
	Glues	61,000	0.2
	Any drug	3,186,000	10.0

*Figures for heroin and crack may be underestimated as the types of groups that use these drugs, e.g. people living in homeless hostels, tend not to overlap with crime survey respondents.
Source: British Crime Survey, 2006/7

9 per cent of 16 to 59 year olds reported having used drugs in the last year, including 2 per cent reporting use of Class A drugs. This rises to 20 per cent and 7 per cent, respectively, for 16 to 24 year olds.

Diagnosis

Diagnosis of drug misuse is usually part of a routine psychiatric assessment or interview. Where a client's drug use is the primary cause for concern a more detailed assessment will be taken, including current and previous drug use, treatments, effects, complications and social history, among other factors. A urine test will be taken and possibly a blood test and the severity of current and possible future problems assessed.

Causes

There is a range of key factors in drug misuse and many may be hidden under other more obvious causes.

Peer group/observation
- Pressure from friends or local role models.
- Vicarious observation of family members using substances.

Age
- People aged 11–24 years are at greatest risk.

Gender
- Males are more susceptible to substance abuse than females.

Availability
- Cost, availability and legal status also affect use.

Other factors
- Iatrogenic factors

- Prescription medicines
- Pleasurable or pharmacological effects
- If the effects are pleasurable or mask reality or pain the substance is more likely to be consumed regularly
- Socioeconomically disadvantaged
- Drugs may be cheap, readily available and provide an 'escape'

Addiction

The addictive quality of a drug is determined by two things – how pleasurable taking the drug is and how quickly the drug reaches the brain. For this reason, drugs that are smoked, injected or snorted can reach the brain very quickly and are usually more addictive than drugs that are swallowed. There is a range of factors, as with other conditions and diseases, that affect addiction traits. These include family history of addiction, a disadvantaged or traumatic childhood, including abuse and neglect, mental health problems, such as depression, anxiety and stress, and an early use of drugs.

In 2007, the medical journal *The Lancet* commissioned drug experts to assess how addictive the most popular misused drugs are and the results were, in order of addictive potential:

- Heroin
- Cocaine
- Tranquilisers
- Amphetamines
- Ketamine
- Cannabis
- Hallucinogens
- Ecstasy

Effects of misuse

A wide range of drugs are misused and new ones become available as others lose popularity. Some of the more common and the broad effects of each 'category' of drug are discussed below (Talk to Frank, 2010).

Short-term effects of drugs

There is a range of pleasant short-term effects of drug misuse and these largely explain the initial use – it feels good. However, many of these effects are fleeting and lead to less pleasant effects which creates a need for more of the substance to relieve the 'come down' or withdrawal symptoms. Hence, the addiction starts with the need to reduce the less pleasant side effects and maintain the desired 'high' for longer (Talk to Frank, 2010).

The long-term physical and psychologial implications of substance misuse are many and vary according to the drug quantity and length of

Stimulants (amphetamines, cocaine, crack)	Hallucinogens (LSD, ecstasy (MDMA) mephedrone (meow meow), phencyclidine (PCP), magic mushrooms)
• Feelings of exhilaration and euphoria • Increased energy and hyperactivity • Rapid or irregular heat beat • Reduced appetite and weight loss • Aggressive or impulsive behaviour • Anxiety or irritability and restlessness • Insomnia • Paranoia • Rapid speech	• Heightened sensory awareness • Hallucinations and euphoria • Impaired perception of reality • Increased heart rate and blood pressure • Nausea and vomiting • Flashbacks, panic or paranoia • Impaired motor function • Memory loss
Opioids/opiates (heroin, methadone, morphine)	Sedatives/hypnotics (benzodiazepines, rohypnol/GHB)
• Euphoria • Drowsiness and sedation • Nausea • Constipation • Confusion • Depression • Depressed respiratory rate	• Drunk in appearance • Balance issues • Speech problems • Amnesia • Delusions • Inability to think clearly or rationally • Increased effect of alcohol
Cannabis (marijuana, weed, skunk)	Volatile substances (solvents/glues, inhalants)
• Sense of relaxation • Heightened sensory awareness • Increase in appetite • Slow thinking and reaction time • Anxiety and paranoia • Impaired coordination • Respiratory problems • Red, dilated eyes • Memory and learning difficulties • Increased heart rate	• Brief 'high' • Loss of inhibition • Headache or • Light-headedness • Nausea or vomiting • Seizures • Impaired motor coordination • Impaired memory • Weakness and fatigue • Risk of sudden death

Figure 2.9 Specific effects of different categories of drug

misuse. However, more common effects include an increased risk of mental health disorders such as paranoia and depression; liver and kidney problems; respiratory problems; cancer; heart problems, e.g. tachycardia, hypertension and cardiovascular disease; depressed or weakened immune system; tremors; cognitive impairment and seizures. Injecting drugs carries the risk of infection at the injection site, endocarditis, septicaemia and transmission of HIV, hepatitis B and C and arterial or venous damage. Drugs that are inhaled or smoked carry greater risks for respiratory or pulmonary complications (Tetrault et al., 2007) as well as additional risks associated with nicotine use.

Nicotine and caffeine

Nicotine

Nicotine is a highly addictive substance and the harmful effects are well documented and evidenced. Although it is strongly associated with mental health problems, it rarely causes them so is not included in this course.

Caffeine

In the DSM-IV-TR, caffeine is classified with cocaine and amphetamines as a central nervous system stimulant. It is widely found in coffee, tea, cocoa, colas and in prescription and over-the-counter pain relief medicine. However, as a CNS stimulant, caffeine, like any other stimulant, has adverse effects when consumed in large quantities.

The DSM-IV-TR lists four disorders relating to excessive caffeine intake; caffeine intoxication, caffeine-induced anxiety disorder, caffeine-induced sleep disorder and caffeine-related disorder not otherwise specified.

While caffeine is an acceptable 'drug' and is not linked with significant addictive properties, it

is estimated that 9–30 per cent of caffeine consumers in the USA may be caffeine-dependent according to DSM criteria for substance dependency. The symptoms of caffeine intoxication include:

- restlessness, nervousness and excitement;
- insomnia;
- facial flushing;
- increased urination;
- gastrointestinal disturbance;
- muscle twitching and/or facial tic;
- talking or thinking in a rambling manner;
- tachycardia;
- periods of inexhaustibility; and/or
- psychomotor agitation.

Treatment interventions in substance misuse

Treatments for substance use and addiction are similar to those for alcohol misuse and include a range of psychological, behavioural and pharmacological interventions.

Residential rehabilitation

This provides the opportunity to be immersed in a positive behaviour situation to help address both the physical dependence and the psychological issues that may have led to the misuse.

Medication

Methadone is used to aid recovery from opioid dependence by providing a controlled and 'clean' alternative to the substance. Buprenorphine is a new pharmacological treatment for opioid dependence. Diazepam is used to reduce non-opioid dependence in gradually decreasing doses over a period of two to six months. For some individuals a maintenance dose may be necessary in the longer term.

Antidepressants may be used to help treat psychological issues that exist alongside misuse of cannabis, ecstasy and inhalants or that arise when the substance is withdrawn.

Nicotine replacement therapy can be helpful in reducing nicotine withdrawal symptoms in the treatment of cannabis dependence.

Therapy/CBT/counselling

The use of various forms of therapy, discussed fully elsewhere in this book, can also help to identify the root problems that may have led to alcohol misuse. The therapy must be chosen to suit the client to have the greatest chance of success.

Motivational interviewing

This technique aims to help a client to move through the stages of change and into action. Discovering the cause of the problem and finding motivation to overcome it are key in recovery. As with smoking cessation, a person needs to want to change their behaviour in order to have a reasonable chance of success. Motivational interviewing is a guiding process led by the client and encourages client responsibility for both the problem and recovery.

Self-help groups like Narcotics Anonymous (NA) can be effective in coping with a substance-related problem and for those who need support from other victims it is a positive route to changing behaviour.

Activity

Physical activity and exercise can be an aid to recovery as they help to fill the gap created by disuse of a substance and distract from withdrawal symptoms and stress, creating a positive behaviour habit. They can also benefit physical health and can help to improve self-esteem and self-efficacy and create a sense of 'health' that has been lacking.

Exercise as intervention in substance misuse

The physical benefits of exercise and activity are well evidenced (BHF, 2009; CMO, 2004) and include improvements to the cardiovascular, respiratory, endocrine, metabolic, gastrointestinal and musculoskeletal systems. In addition the psychological benefits, particularly those relating to depression, stress and anxiety, are well documented.

There is a lack of research into the benefits of using activity as an aid to treatment interventions in substance misuse, mainly due to the individual nature of treatment making any controlled trials difficult. There are also many factors plus a risk of relapse that also make any comparison difficult. However, the research that exists does indicate a positive relationship with cessation (Biddle & Mutrie, 2001).

However, there is a considerable amount of research into activity and nicotine cessation that may be transferrable in part to substance misuse cessation. In a key paper, Bess found that when exercise was included as part of a treatment intervention in nicotine cessation the exercise group had twice the successful quit rate than those who did not exercise (Bess et al.,1999:1229–1234). The report also discussed research on rats and found that rats that had access to a running wheel had a lower consumption of amphetamines – perhaps due to the endorphin high triggered by activity. Furthermore, research carried out in 1995 and 2010 concluded that increased physical activity levels were associated with decreased use of tobacco and marijuana and increased participation in health-promoting behaviours in teenagers (Scott et al., 1995; Delisle et al., 2010:134–140).

There are also benefits from outdoor activities such as walking, gardening, conservation work and rambling as the natural environment has a strong influence on an individual's relationship with 'place', which can help to create a sense of coherence and decrease feelings of confusion and anxiety. The natural environment, particularly that with trees, is consistently a preferred location for individuals with mental health issues and is therefore important in creating a sense of belonging and identity, which in turn improves mental health (Bird, 2007).

Programming activity or exercise will need to take into account many factors and allow for improvements that are more gradual in fitness, however, the distraction provided may be the biggest benefit. Many anecdotal accounts report that the time out, distraction or just being around others and doing something is the main attraction of exercise.

The obstacles

As with any drugs, both legally prescribed and illicit, there are side effects that may have an impact on exercise ability and tolerance. Long term, or even short term, use of a drug, substance or alcohol can affect the function of the central nervous system and impair motor nerve function. Long-term substance abuse can cause peripheral vasodilation and increased heat loss that can affect strength and speed of muscle contraction. Alcohol in particular affects muscles, causing inflammation

and possible cell death that affects both muscle strength and endurance and peripheral neuropathy may be present which can influence balance and coordination.

Activity participation is further complicated by the long-term effects of negative lifestyles and health perceptions typical of individuals with severe mental illness or long-term addictions (Crone, 2004:19–25). There may be further obstacles from cognitive or psychological impairments including inability to focus, memory loss, lethargy and depression that can prove to be more significant barriers to activity than physical factors.

In general, whatever the physical outcome, exercise and activity are welcome additions to treatment plans as they provide a focus and distraction from the condition, thoughts and withdrawal symptoms and can also encourage social interaction and a chance to chat.

Dual diagnosis

Dual diagnosis is a term used with individuals with a mental health problem who also misuse drugs or alcohol. It is an important diagnosis as it highlights that there may be additional difficulties experienced by the individual, not necessarily medical or psychological, but relating to lifestyle matters such as housing, welfare and legal issues.

It is estimated that between 30 and 50 per cent of people with a mental health problem also have issues with drug or alcohol misuse, rising to over 50 per cent of those in secure units. Additionally, between half and two-thirds of people who are treated for drug or alcohol problems may have a mental health condition.

The use of drugs or alcohol are linked with mental health conditions in three ways. They can:

- directly cause mental health problems (e.g. stimulants such as amphetamines and cocaine);
- aggravate mental health problems (e.g. cannabis, LSD, ecstasy and opiates); and
- be used to relieve mental health problems (e.g. alcohol).

Additionally, taking two or more drugs simultaneously can change the way they react causing toxicity or an increase or decrease in the treatment effect of prescribed medication. This is particularly true of 'street' drugs that may be mixed with unknown ingredients that can lead to significant adverse effects.

In the past this has been a difficult diagnosis to treat as the individual may have a chaotic lifestyle, however the use of interventions such as motivational interviewing, family therapy and the 12-step approaches used by organisations like Alcoholics Anonymous may be helpful.

SUMMARY POINTS

You should now be able to:

- List the range of classified mental health conditions discussed.
- State the signs and symptoms of:
  - Schizophrenia
  - Bipolar disorder
  - Depression
  - Stress
  - GAD
  - Anorexia nervosa
  - Bulimia nervosa.
- Describe the effects of each condition on physiological systems (neurological, muscular skeletal, CV, respiratory, endocrine).
- Explain some comorbidities that may exist with specific mental health conditions (obesity, high blood pressure, COPD, other mental health conditions, etc.).
- Describe factors which may contribute to the development of each condition.
- Suggest a range of interventions and treatments for each condition.
- State some of the physiological effects of different medications used to treat specific mental health conditions.

THE BENEFITS OF EXERCISE

3

The benefits of exercise and physical activity are well documented. This chapter will review some of the benefits and guide you towards legislation reporting these benefits. Also reviewed are some of the theoretical hypotheses linked between exercise and mental health, giving reference to sources for further reading and research. The barriers to exercise for persons with mental health conditions are explored, with preliminary suggestions for promoting participation and adherence.

OBJECTIVES

By the end of this section you should be able to:

*   recognise the benefits of exercise for improving mental and physical health;
*   recognise the recommended physical activity targets to improve fitness and health;
*   recognise the long term physiological adaptations from exercise and physical activity;
*   recognise barriers to exercise faced by persons with mental health conditions; and
*   recognise strategies for health promotion.

THE CASE FOR EXERCISE

The physical health benefits of regular activity and exercise participation are well known and publicised. They include improved cardiovascular fitness, increased muscular strength and endurance, better flexibility, mobility, motor skills and balance plus an overall sense of well-being. Additional benefits include improved eating patterns leading to weight loss and weight management, which can help to improve body image and self-esteem.

Equally well documented are the benefits for 'medical' health, including decreased risk factors for a range of conditions including heart disease, osteoporosis, hypertension, obesity, arthritis, diabetes and cancer.

When it comes to mental health the 'feel better' benefit of exercise is also well known, yet the number of people active enough to benefit both their physical and mental health has remained relatively static at around 30 per cent for over a decade (Health Survey for England, 2008).

In recent years, several government white papers have highlighted the growing awareness of the role of lifestyle as an initial or additional form of prevention and treatment for mental health problems.

- **Saving Lives: Our Healthier Nation:** Published in 1999, this identified mental health as a key area for development leading to awareness of the role of an integrative approach to prevention and treatment in both primary and secondary care.
- **The NICE guidelines for the treatment of depression (2004)** state that, 'Patients of all ages with mild depression should be advised of the benefits of following a structured and supervised exercise programme of typically up to three sessions a week of moderate duration (45 minutes to 1 hour) for between 10 and 12 weeks'.
- **The Chief Medical Officer report (2004)** states that, 'Physical activity is effective in the treatment of clinical depression and can be as successful as psychotherapy or medication, particularly in the longer term'.
- **The Department of Health (in 'Making it happen** – A guide to delivering mental health promotion', 2001) states that, 'Physical activity is emerging as an effective treatment for directly tackling existing mental health problems' and, 'Physical activity has a comparable level of effect on depression as that obtained from psychotherapeutic interventions'.

These initiatives and reports aim to promote activity and exercise as a pro-active strategy to help reduce the economic burden of medical problems on the NHS, with a specific mental health-related aim to reduce the death rate from suicide and undetermined injury by at least one-fifth by 2010.

EXERCISE AND MENTAL HEALTH – THE EVIDENCE

There is a plethora of research to show that exercise and activity has both a short-term (acute) and long-term (chronic) effect on depression, particularly when used in conjunction with a talking therapy. Key research is discussed in the Mental Health Foundation (MHF) report 'Up and Running' published in April 2005, which looked at the attitudes of GPs towards depression and treatments and concluded that it is a lack of awareness about exercise as therapy rather than refusal to refer that is the main barrier to referral for exercise.

Levels of tension and paranoia are decreased and a sense of mastery and self-efficacy are increased with long-term regular exercise. Other reported benefits include feeling happier and more satisfied with life and an increase in self-worth and self-image. The benefits of activity on mental health state appear to be greater in at-risk groups such as young women, young offenders and those from black and minority ethnic groups.

Health benefits are also significant, as depression usually coexists with significantly low fitness levels due to the sedentary effects of the condition, which increases the risk factors for many physical conditions such as diabetes, obesity and cardiovascular disease. There does not appear to be a significant difference in benefits between CV or MSE exercise, although weight training does appear to improve self-esteem in men. What is significant is adherence to exercise appears to be the key to the treatment factor and, with over half of patients continuing to exercise regularly in the long term and a better ongoing success rate than therapy, it needs to be more widely prescribed.

QUALITY OF LIFE

Exercise and activity are also promoted as ways to improve quality of life. However, 'quality of life' is a multidimensional concept relating to a set of values that are unique to each organism, person or context.

The more complex or developed the organism becomes, so the values or criteria for determining fitness or quality of life become linearly complex.

In order to evaluate quality of life many factors must be taken into account including the effect of outside influences on an individual together with the changing inner physical and mental structure. There are also different levels of effect, especially with regard to medications. It is often the case that a medication can have a beneficial effect on a physical or mental condition but can cause damage to other cells. For example, steroids are effective in the long term control of asthma but damage bones, while atypical antipsychotics help stabilise mental states and control the symptoms of schizophrenia but affect metabolism adversely, leading to weight gain.

Quality of life therefore is not merely the absence of internal disease or disorders or external environmental hazards but takes into account more fluid, changing aspects of life and existence both internal and external. The higher increase in salary for someone moving from a rural environment to a city may not be seen to compensate for the perceived better standard of living currently enjoyed. Thus, the term 'quality of life' when applied to the benefits of regular activity may be a subjective or qualitative measure of an individual's physical and mental state rather than a quantitative one, although it is still valid.

EXERCISE OR MEDICATION?

Hopefully the aforementioned government guidelines and the evidence for exercise will lead to more people being offered exercise as an initial treatment for mild and moderate depression, anxiety and stress, or as an additional treatment alongside medication.

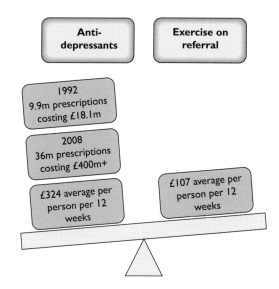

Figure 3.1 The cost of anti-depressants vs. the cost of exercise on prescription (adapted from MHF, 'Up and Running', 2005)

Medication for mental illness makes up one-quarter of the total prescriptions issued within the NHS and the cost is considerable so any intervention that helps to reduce this economic burden should be welcomed.

In an evaluation of their exercise referral scheme, South Tyneside produced the following figures relating to the cost of exercise on referral versus medication.

A survey by the mental health charity Mind (2001) highlighted the importance of exercise and activity for both therapeutic and preventative finding that:

- 83 per cent of people with mental health problems have used physical activity and exercise to help lift their mood/reduce stress.
- 75 per cent of gym members used exercise to reduce stress.

- 68 per cent of gym members thought their general mental well-being would suffer if they stopped exercising.
- 65 per cent of people with mental health problems said exercise had helped to relieve depressive symptoms, while figures for symptom relief of other conditions are also high (62 per cent stress, 56 per cent anxiety, 12 per cent manic depression, 10 per cent schizophrenia).
- 57 per cent of people with mental health problems reported improved motivation from being active, 50 per cent improved self-esteem, 24 per cent improved social skills.
- 35 per cent of gym members reported improved performance at work.

Medication is unquestionably appropriate for some mental health disorders, particularly the more severe conditions and for some people it is, literally, a lifesaver. However, exercise as an initial treatment for less severe cases may be as effective and it carries none of the side effects (apart from occasional muscle soreness!).

In the short term, though, medication may bring about enough relief from symptoms to enable the individual to become more active and benefit from both medication and the effects of exercise, so the dual treatment approach may be useful.

BENEFITS OF EXERCISE AND PHYSICAL ACTIVITY FOR MENTAL HEALTH

Ryan (1984) in Leith (1995) reports that the forefather of medicine, Hippocrates, prescribed exercise to patients with mental illness. However, Leith (1995:3) indicates that any large-scale research on the area of exercise and mental health

has been thwarted by the dualistic approach to exercise and mental health promoted by the medical model. Only a few professional and academic schools of physical education, therapeutic recreation and psychosomatic medicine continue the research and interest in this area (Dishman, 1986, in Leith, 1994).

However, over the last two decades, there has been a substantial interest and evidence base to support the role of physical activity for managing both medical and mental health. These include:

- The government white paper *Saving Lives: Our Healthier Nation* (1999) which cited mental health as one of the four main areas to be targeted regionally and locally for strategic development.
- *National Service Framework: Mental Health* (1999)
- *NHS Plan* (2000)
- *The National Quality Assurance Framework: Exercise Referral Systems* (2001)
- *Chief Medical Officer Annual Report: The State of Public Health* (2009)
- *Tackling Health Inequalities: A Programme for Action* (2003)
- *Choosing Health* (CMO, 2004)
- *At Least Five a Week* (CMO, 2005)
- *Fulfilled Lives, Supportive Communities: Social Service Reform* (2007)
- *No Health without Mental Health* (2011)

The messages regarding the benefits of physical activity are numerous and clearly evidenced in all CMO reports which state that physically active adults have:

- improved psychological well-being;

- reduced risk of clinical depression, stress and anxiety;
- 20–30 per cent reduced risk of premature death;
- up to 50 per cent reduced risk of diseases such as coronary heart disease (CHD), stroke, diabetes and certain cancers;
- improved functional capacity;
- reduced risk of back pain;
- increased independence (older people);
- increased bone density and reduced risk of osteoporosis;
- reduced risk of falls (older adults); and
- improved weight loss and weight management.

In his report of 2009 on the state of public health, Sir Liam Donaldson, the then-Chief Medical Officer for the Department for Health, stated:

'The health and wider benefits of physical activity are substantial. If a medication existed that decreased the risks of chronic disease to a comparable extent, it would undoubtedly become one of the most widely prescribed drugs within the NHS. As a population, we can harness all of these benefits by taking simple and inexpensive steps to become more active. The scourge of inactivity has been ignored for too long. This is the time for action.' (Department of Health (DoH), 2009:28)

PHYSICAL ACTIVITY AND HEALTH PROMOTION

As discussed, physical activity features in many government policies and initiatives as a medium for improving and promoting health.

RECOMMENDED MINIMUM LEVELS OF PHYSICAL ACTIVITY FOR ADULTS

The current recommendations for minimum levels of physical activity to maintain general health are set out in the *Strategy Statement on*

Table 3.1	Department of Health targets for physical activity
Frequency	Work towards building activity into daily routine on 5 days of the week (minimum)
Intensity	Work at a moderate level where you feel mildly breathless, warm but comfortable (level 3–4 on the adapted RPE intensity scale in section 8)
Time	Work towards performing the chosen activities for a total of 30 minutes. This can be broken down and accumulated, for example: 3 x 10 minute slots of activity or 2 x 15 minute slots of activity a day
Type	Any activity that fits well into your daily lifestyle, for example: • Walking to the station/school • Vigorous housework • Cleaning the car • Using stairs more frequently • Dancing to music at home • Active hobbies • Structured exercise and sporting activities • A combination of activity, exercise and sport This recommendation can be tailored specifically to the lifestyle, preference and needs of the individual and is particularly relevant for the people who find it easier and more acceptable to increase physical activity by incorporating it into their everyday life.

Physical Activity by the Department of Health (1996 and 2005) and the ACSM (2007). These targets are outlined in table 3.1.

These guidelines are currently under review in light of more recent evidence from the USA. Evidence from the USA indicates that a total volume of 150 minutes of physical activity should be accumulated over a week, but can be spread over the week in a variety of ways. A further suggestion is that persons involved in more vigorous exercise, could work towards a lower volume of 75 minutes per week (Source: DoH, CMO report, 2009, U.S. Department of Health and Human Services, 2008). These guidelines are formed from a scientific literature review relating to several characteristics of physical activity and impact on health outcomes. Full information can be found at www.health.gov/PAGuidelines/Report.

ANATOMICAL AND PHYSIOLOGICAL ADAPTATIONS TO EXERCISE

There are numerous longer term adaptations from specific types of exercise that improve our daily functioning.

CARDIOVASCULAR TRAINING

Low cardiovascular fitness is associated with an increased risk of chronic diseases such as diabetes, high blood pressure, high cholesterol and coronary heart disease, all of which ultimately cause pre-mature death.

Regular cardiovascular exercise enables many beneficial anatomical and physiological adaptations that improve health. This includes improved heart and lung function, which leads to better pulmonary and muscular capillary networks to allow transportation of more oxygen to the cells and swifter removal of waste products and an increase in the size and number of mitochondria, enabling increased utilisation of oxygen.

FLEXIBILITY TRAINING

Being able to move the joints and muscles through their full potential range of movement is essential for easing the performance of all of our everyday tasks and maintaining independence. A full range of movement also helps with posture as muscles that are too loose or tight will create muscular imbalances and affect posture.

MUSCULAR FITNESS TRAINING

Muscles need to be strong enough and have sufficient endurance to carry out daily tasks, which require lifting, carrying, pulling or pushing a resistance. This includes carrying shopping, gardening, moving furniture, climbing stairs and lifting the body to/from a chair or into/out of a bath. Strong muscles help to maintain the correct skeletal alignment as weakened muscles may cause an uneven pull on the skeleton. Muscles work in pairs (as one contracts and works, the opposite muscle relaxes) so any imbalance in workload will cause joints to be pulled out of correct alignment. This may potentially cause injury, or create postural defects such as rounded shoulders or excessive curvatures of the spine (lordosis, kyphosis, scoliosis, flatback, swayback, winged scapula, etc.).

Muscular fitness training improves muscle tone and function and provides a firmer and shapelier appearance which can contribute to a positive self-image and enhance psychological well-being and self-confidence.

Muscular fitness also improves the strength and health of bones and joints. The contraction of muscles pulls against the bones to create movement and in response, the tendons (attaching the muscles to bone across the joint) and ligaments (attaching bone to bone across the joint) will become stronger. This results in stronger, more stable joints, which are at less risk from injury. In addition, this stress on the bones results in increased calcium deposition and storage in the bones which helps reduce the risk of osteoporosis. Muscular fitness training can therefore provide many long-lasting benefits, which can extend quality of life for a number of years.

Motor fitness can have a direct effect on functional ability and an indirect effect on the ability to function in the other components of fitness. Development of specific skills such as speed and coordination can improve performance of everyday activities and enable more skilful movement and safer exercise techniques. This helps to reduce the risk of injury and will maximise both the safety and effectiveness of performance.

Managing body weight, coordinating body movements and moving at different speeds, in different directions and at different intensities, will also contribute to improving our motor fitness.

PHYSIOLOGICAL ADAPTATIONS DURING EXERCISE

The body adapts physiologically in numerous ways during exercise. Some of these physical adaptations have been researched and reported as having a positive effect on psychological well-being. These include:

- increased heart rate and circulation leading to an increased core and muscle temperature which can provide a short-term relaxing effect similar to a warm bath;
- enhanced neurotransmission of chemicals released by the endocrine system (norepinephrine, serotonin and dopamine), which lead to improvements in mood;
- improved circulation of endorphins, contributing to the 'feel good factor' being experienced;
- increased adrenal activity, leading to increased steroid reserves, which can potentially offer an increased ability to cope with stressful situations more effectively;
- energy expenditure increases providing a physical release for increased glucose in the circulatory system caused by the 'fight or flight' response;

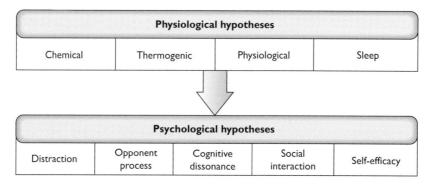

Figure 3.2 An overview of theoretical models

- increased mental focus and concentration, which offers a distraction from other thoughts and can provide a sense of balance and perspective to anxieties and concerns; and/or
- muscle work offering a release from increased muscle tension caused by the stress response 'fight or flight'.

THE RELATIONSHIP BETWEEN EXERCISE AND MENTAL HEALTH

There are various schools of thought about the mechanisms of how exercise benefits mental health and the key hypotheses are:

PHYSIOLOGICAL HYPOTHESES
The chemical hypothesis

This looks at the actions of two chemicals in the brain, monoamines and endorphins. The endorphin theory proposes that exercise causes the release of chemicals called endorphins and enkephalin, a subunit of endorphins, which are the body's natural pain killer (similar to morphine) and are often cited as responsible for the 'feel good factor' and feeling of euphoria that many report they experience through exercise.

'Endurance running produces a marked increase in beta endorphin. Whether this increase persists after physical activity and is responsible for the runner's high, the behavioural alterations of endurance trained individuals, improved libido, heightened pain threshold, absence of depression and other anecdotal effects of endurance training remains conjectural.' Appenzeller et al., in Leith (1994:7).

However, despite anecdotal evidence, there is still limited scientific evidence to actually prove the hypothesis. Leith (1994:7) provides an overview of a number of different investigations and suggests that Appenzeller et al. (1980:149) provide a useful summary of the collective research so far.

Monoamine theory

The basis of this theory is that exercise has a normalising effect on the balance of neurotransmitters (primarily monoamine chemicals including serotonin, noradrenalin and dopamine) in the brain. These chemicals have been linked with mental health conditions and are found in lower concentrations in individuals with depression. Some researchers suggest that the improved affect from exercise is due to changes in these chemicals.

Again, there is no absolute or conclusive evidence, however Leith (1994:10) suggests that based on the reviews of a number of researchers (Biddle & Fox, 1989; D.R. Brown, 1990; Dienstbier, 1989; Johnsgard, 1989; Morgan, 1988; Riggs, 1991 and Sime, 1990) there is significant reason to 'speculate a monoamine relationship between exercise and mental health,' (Leith 1994:10).

Neuroendocrine changes brought on by exercise are believed to increase the efficiency of the adrenal glands and improve the physiological response to stress. In addition, exercise may bring on changes that are associated with a relaxed state such as relaxed muscles, physical tiredness and a sense of achievement.

Thermogenic hypothesis

This is one of the most enduring theories and is based on the premise that an increase in body temperature due to increased activity leads to health improvements, as when the body temperature is elevated (e.g. during exercise, hot baths, saunas, etc.) the body is more relaxed. This reaction is similar to the immune response that raises body temperature to kill off invaders. Research appears to link this effect with anxiety rather than depression (DeVries, 1981).

Physiological adaptations

Regular activity promotes a number of physiological benefits including improved body composition leading to a better body image, release of tension, normalisation of blood pressure, as well as all the physical benefits mentioned earlier (Hamer, 2010). Furthermore, looking better makes you feel better.

Improved sleep

Better sleep patterns can bring about major improvements in both physical and psychological states. The old saying 'everything looks better after a good night's sleep' is very true and regular exercisers demonstrate improvements in both length and quality of sleep (Biddles, SJH 2001: 198).

PSYCHOLOGICAL HYPOTHESES
Distraction

Distraction plays a role in helping to control negative thinking due to the need to concentrate on what one is doing rather than thinking – a sort of mental 'time out'. Many people report that exercise provides an opportunity to forget about the condition or the effects of the condition and have some time for the self and offers a distraction to stressful situations we may experience.

The area that needs to be addressed in future research would be to compare the effects of exercise as opposed to other past times – knitting, reading, watching TV, gardening, etc. to confirm whether the exercise or the distraction is the key (Leith, 1994:12).

Self-efficacy

The sense of achievement when an exercise session is completed successfully leads to improved self-efficacy and a more 'can do' way of thinking. This can lead to a decrease in anxiety as the sense of 'self' and ability improves.

Social interaction

Social isolation is common in the daily life of an individual with a mental health disorder so any form of group activity that increases social contact is important for a sense of belonging, and attending a regular session can add structure to the day.

The opponent-process model of acquired motivation

Leith (1994) suggests this model is unique in that it uses a physiological mechanism (e.g. endorphins) to explain a psychological change; the assumption being 'that the brain is organised to oppose pleasurable or aversive emotional processes' (Leith 1994:12). The key premise is that when the body is aroused by a stimulus (e.g. exercise) there is increased sympathetic nervous system activity (all physiological responses 'speed up') and in response, the body will produce a counter response (opponent) to maintain homeostasis (e.g. relaxation – or slowing down, via parasympathetic nervous system activity) and longevity of exposure to the stimulus (exercise) will bring about a stronger opponent response (relaxation) which is believed to responsible for the positive benefits to mental health. In simpler terms, the body will do what it can to keep itself in balance. Leith (1994) guides to the research of Petruzzello et al., (1991) for further information.

Cognitive dissonance theory

Cognitive dissonance occurs when an individual holds conflicting beliefs. The theory evolves from the work of Festinger, 1957. Petruzzello et al., (1991) in Leith (1994:13) suggests that in order to feel good after exercise, 'people who continue to exercise have to find a way to justify their exercise behaviour, thereby overcoming the initial negative effect of exercise' for example, exercise can be uncomfortable, it demands effort and exertion and the initial getting started phase is not pleasant (breathless, hot, sweaty, muscles start working and aching etc.), so to keep going, one has to remind themselves mentally that it is good for them, that they will feel better afterwards – shifting both attitude and mood towards a more positive frame. There is no scientific evidence to support this theory.

NB: It should be noted that research is ongoing and these theories are only an introduction to some of the available literature.

BARRIERS TO BEING MORE ACTIVE

Most people build barriers to keep exercise or activity at bay. 71 per cent of the population are not active enough to benefit their health and nearly one-quarter do less than 20 minutes of moderate activity a week. Figure 3.3 shows just some of the excuses used to justify a lack of activity.

The key reason is often fear: Fear of looking foolish; not coping; being the fattest/least fit/oldest; not keeping up and the overriding sense that 'I can't do it'. This sense of 'can't' usually dictates the outcome so one of the biggest challenges is to show an individual that they 'can'.

Barriers or blocks to being more active can be classified as either **intrinsic** or **extrinsic**. Intrinsic barriers relate to how the individual feels about physical activity. This will be influenced by their past experiences (school, family experience, etc.) and their beliefs concerning physical activity (education, family, socialisation, etc.) which can influence both interest in physical activity and confidence to take part in physical activities. For example, 'I am not a sporty person, I don't like exercising, I'm no good at exercising, I'm too fat to go to a gym or exercise class, I'm not fit enough, I'm too embarrassed to go to a gym or exercise class, I'm too tired to exercise, etc.'

Extrinsic barriers relate to broader issues such as access to and availability of appropriate and affordable physical activity (e.g. leisure centres, community centres, activity groups), the environment (e.g. roads, parks, concerns for personal safety), opportunities for physical activity (work, school, home) and the attitude and skills of other people (exercise professionals, family, teachers, health professionals, etc.). For example, 'I don't have time, there aren't any facilities close to where I live, my family need me, I need to relax after working all day, I cannot afford to join a gym, I cannot afford to buy exercise clothing or pay for a weekly exercise session, etc.'

The Department of Health (2005) and Health Development Agency (2005) reports both cite other social factors that influence participation in sport and exercise. They indicate lower levels of

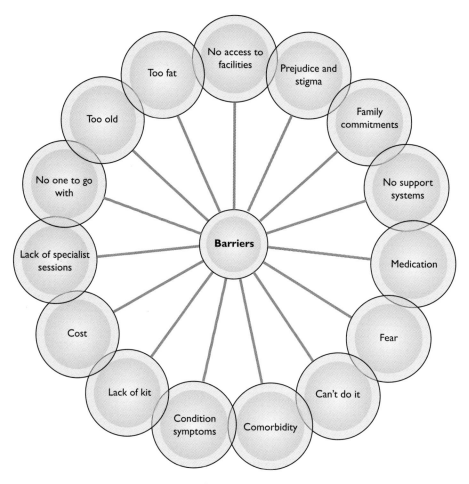

Figure 3.3 Barriers to exercise

physical activity reported among the following populations:

- Some minority ethnic groups
- People in low income households
- Lower social classes
- People with lower levels of educational attainment
- People performing non-professional and non-managerial status work

- Older people

Older people and people with other medical conditions may face additional barriers, which include:

- Fear of overdoing it
- Fear of injuring themselves or aggravating a medical condition
- Feeling they don't fit in or wouldn't be able to keep up

- Safety fears, such as a fear of falling in some environments (e.g. swimming pools)
- Lack of culturally appropriate facilities

Source: *Active for Later Life*, BHF (2003)

The list of potential and perceived barriers is endless, and arguably, most of these can be viewed as self-made excuses for maintaining current behaviour and lifestyle patterns. However, if the individual views these as barriers that are 'real' for them, then these barriers should be considered carefully and sensitively by the exercise professional and discussed with the client before an exercise programme is prescribed or recommended.

MENTAL ILL-HEALTH BARRIERS
Mental ill-health potentially provides one of the greatest barriers to regular participation in exercise and physical activity. People diagnosed with depression find it hard to engage in their regular daily routine, often struggling to find the motivation to complete basic daily activities such as self-care (getting out of bed, getting dressed) and home care (housework, food preparation and cooking). Consequently, taking part in hobbies or other previously enjoyed interests will have much less appeal, as their ability to find enjoyment and purpose from these activities is temporarily lost. In addition, some mental health conditions affect the ability to experience pleasure. It becomes harder to find enjoyment in being active or to see beyond the experience of the condition from which they are suffering at that time. It may also be difficult to focus and concentrate on tasks, and sufferers therefore become distracted more easily.

These factors, combined with the feelings of hopelessness, futility and inadequacy that are frequently experienced by persons with mental health conditions, will create further barriers. Low levels of self-esteem and confidence, a lack of belief in self-worth and negative associations about ability and body image will provide further barriers that contribute to both a lack of energy and desire to be active.

MEDICATION AS A BARRIER
The side effects from some medications may provide a further barrier, as they can impair the individual's ability and capacity to exercise.

There are a wide range of side effects that have implications for exercise (see box) and these need to be considered when planning a session. Cardiovascular issues such as arrhythmias and

Side effects of medication

CV issues: Arrhythmias, tachycardia, hypertension, syncope, postural hypotension, palpitations

Musculoskeletal issues: Movement disorders, arthralgia, myalgia, tremor

CNS issues: Confusion, sedation, blurred vision, sweating, convulsions, light-headedness, vertigo, dizziness

Other issues: Angioedema, paraesthesia, hypomania, mania, urinary retention, constipation, dry mouth, gastro-intestinal disorders, insomnia, drowsiness, increased sweating

NB: Other medication creates side effects that need consideration when planning the intensity, duration and type of exercise recommended, and the method selected to monitor intensity (e.g. beta-blockers prescribed for anxiety).

palpitations necessitate a longer warm-up and cool down while musculoskeletal issues such as arthralgia (joint pain) and myalgia (muscle pain) indicate a need for lower intensity and impact.

PHYSICAL FITNESS AND SYMPTOM BARRIERS

Individuals with mental health conditions may have lower fitness than expected. This is potentially one of the greatest barriers to being more active, especially if they have not experienced the benefits of regular activity or exercise in the past. In addition, different mental health conditions present specific signs and symptoms that may raise barriers:

- **Anxiety problems:** Increased heart rate and breathlessness
- **Panic disorders** may be triggered by being in specific environments (e.g. in crowds or travelling)
- **Phobias:** Fears associated with experiencing increased body temperature, sweating, increased heart rate and breathing rate, flushing (the immediate physiological response to exercise) are all symptoms of their condition and may cause additional distress to them
- **OCD:** Cleanliness and touching may present barriers, such as using mats or equipment used by others for fear of contamination
- **Depressive phases:** Psychomotor retardation (the slowing down of thoughts and physical movements), low motivation and lethargy
- **Manic episodes:** Psychomotor agitation (restlessness brought on by muscle tension), inability to concentrate and psychosis
- **Catatonic schizophrenia:** Clumsiness, stiffness of joints or stiffness of movement

SOCIAL SUPPORT BARRIERS

Mental health conditions often lead to a person withdrawing from social environments. This may contribute to communication difficulties, fear of being in the company of others and anxiety when in social situations. Low self-esteem and confidence, previous negative experiences of exercising, fear of the unknown and inaccurate expectations or beliefs about exercise, coupled with a fear of being around people who are 'fitness experts', will compound these fears.

Another social barrier is having a lack of support or understanding from family or friends. People can often lack empathy around people with mental health conditions and consequently are not able to be comfortable in their company. Many people find it much easier to be active and make changes if they have a training partner or a person or group to support them with their planned changes (e.g. Alcoholics Anonymous).

Social barriers are compounded if the client is unable to access support from a person who speaks their native language. This includes the availability of information and resources they can access for finding help in the first place. This raises the issue for specific support resources being available in different languages.

ENVIRONMENTAL BARRIERS – FACILITIES AND EQUIPMENT

Some regions have reduced access to facilities or would require the person to travel a greater distance to access these facilities. These barriers are increased if the person has a phobia or fear of travelling to or accessing facilities.

In addition, the equipment in gyms may be intimidating for some people with mental health conditions as it can appear complex to operate.

Entering personal data to programme cardio-vascular machines may further demotivate a depressed client and also increase anxiety.

QUALIFIED FITNESS PROFESSIONAL BARRIERS

A lack of skilled and qualified fitness professionals with experience of working with this population creates a further barrier. To promote adherence to activity, any sessions must accurately reflect the abilities and needs of the individual and the fitness professional needs to understand the barriers that may be experienced to plan appropriate exercise. Any limitations or lack of support for people with mental health problems will compound their fears and create further potential barriers to activity.

Exercise professionals who would like to work with persons with mental health disorders must ensure they are free from their own prejudices and can be empathic and non-judgmental towards the individual. They also need to be able to identify support and supervision systems, both in and out of the work place that can assist them when working with this particular group. Working with clients with mental health conditions can be challenging and can often raise personal issues to the surface. Counsellors are required to undertake one hour of supervision (when they completed a set number of client work hours, e.g. every six clients) on a regular basis to support their client work; they may also at times have to enter personal therapy to work through their own issues. Exercise professionals could use the services of counsellors and other mental health professionals to support their work. This support service is more likely to be available and considered in a professional health setting working with persons with mental health conditions, rather than at the local sports centre). Working towards and maintaining mental health is a lifelong journey and it is essential that this is supported by the appropriate professionals.

RISKS ASSOCIATED WITH HEALTH-RELATED PHYSICAL ACTIVITY

The benefits of physical activity are substantial and far outweigh the risks associated with participation. Many of the risks associated with physical activity are avoidable through appropriate initial risk assessment procedures, discussed in part 3. At risk groups would include people who:

- do too much exercise;
- want to take part in vigorous activity or competitive sport;
- do too much too soon; and/or
- have an existing condition or disease which may require an adapted programme.

People who do too much exercise are rare; however there are individuals who become obsessive about exercise. For example, people with eating disorders such as anorexia nervosa may use exercise as a way to control their weight. They will experience withdrawal symptoms if they are prevented from exercising. This obsessive behaviour is not caused by exercise, but is more likely to be connected to an underlying psychological disorder and/or may be an addictive tendency within the personality.

PROMOTING PARTICIPATION

There are numerous strategies that need to be considered to promote participation.

ACCESS AND INCLUSION

Many local health services are engaged with promoting activity for mental health. It is useful to find out who the key stakeholders (mental health charities, public health organisations, local and national government etc.) are in your area and make contact with them to offer your services as a fitness professional. Funding opportunities to reduce the cost of exercise and activity sessions may also be available.

Small groups with less severe mental health conditions can go to an exercise facility to take part in a specific programme. This can help to increase their confidence in social situations and may enhance social reintegration. The fitness professional will need to make contact with leisure providers to promote this service and, if necessary, break down the prejudice attached to mental health.

UNIT-/SERVICE-BASED SESSIONS

Taking exercise to the service users by setting up an exercise session within a mental health facility is another way of making activity and exercise more accessible. Some specialist services such as physiotherapy or occupational therapy teams working in mental health will employ a fitness professional to deliver this facility within their service. Other services (mental health charities etc.) will rely on the availability of funding or 'goodwill' to enable this service to be provided. Part of the assessment for the level 4 physical activity for persons with mental health conditions requires exercise professional to find a placement where they can work with service users and be supported by other health professionals (supervised practice). This may be a voluntary placement or it may be an employed placement. The intention

is that this will enable activity and exercise to be more widely available, create potential work opportunities and even attract funding and support to meet the objectives listed on the recent government strategy paper – no health without mental health.

Service-based programmes offer an opportunity for users to become familiar with the different types of exercise and activity available and individuals can be encouraged to observe sessions before taking part. They can also meet the fitness professional and other participants, which can provide a bridge between inactivity and non-participation to activity and participation.

Running exercise programmes in conjunction with specific support groups run by other organisations (MIND, Alcoholics Anonymous, etc.) also offers potential for taking exercise to the population, rather than demanding they find their way to exercise. As with sessions run in mental health units, the advantage is that the participants are in familiar 'safe' surroundings which help reduce any anxiety that may be felt.

INVOLVING OTHER HEALTH PROFESSIONALS IN EXERCISE REFERRAL SCHEMES

Involving other medical and health professionals as well as GPs is another way of promoting participation. Medical professionals can be very influential over clients so a recommendation to be more active or take part in an exercise programme may have more credibility. There are a small number of exercise on referral schemes available throughout the UK. One of the most successful programmes is the National Exercise Referral

Scheme (NERS) funded by the Welsh Assembly Government, which operates throughout the whole of Wales. Clients are referred to the programme by their GP and undertake a physical and health assessment by a qualified professional, they are then entered into a programme of supervised exercise for a specified time period; from which their progress is reviewed and other opportunities for activity may be introduced (exit routes to general and appropriate mainstream sessions) if appropriate. Also the individual may have greater trust in the fitness professional's competence if they are referred by someone they recognise as qualified. The Register of Exercise professionals (REPs) are now working closely with other health professionals to encourage the recognition of exercise as part of a treatment plan to improve health. REPs have a list of all instructors who have achieved specific qualifications in specialist areas.

SESSION STRUCTURE AND DESIGN

All sessions should be simple, fun and generally less complex and less intense and for a shorter duration, depending on the specific group and individual and the condition they present. Any physical activity programme should be aimed to improve the self-efficacy of the client – shaming and blaming for not being fit enough or not being able to perform certain exercises would be inappropriate.

Ways to motivate and encourage include:

- offering praise to the person for turning up – even if they only want to sit and watch the first session)
- remaining engaged with them throughout by asking if they want to join in specific components of the session (e.g. how about trying this relaxation activity or asking them to offer praise and encouragement to others)
- making them feel welcome – when they are taking part, providing positive encouragement etc.

DRESS AND ATTIRE

The perceived image of the super-fit exercise professional clad in the latest kit can be avoided if the fitness professional dresses in a more conservative style. Selected dress code and attire should be respectful to different religions, cultures and/or sexual beliefs and/or adhere to unit policy (where appropriate).

Participants may not have all the latest fitness gear and attire, so it is advisable to allow them to participate wearing the clothing they feel most comfortable in. Provided this does not present a health and safety risk, their chosen outfit should be accepted.

SUMMARY POINTS

You should now be able to:

- List some of the benefits of exercise and activity for improving mental and physical health.
- State the recommended physical activity targets to improve fitness and health.
- List some of the long-term physiological adaptations gained from taking part in exercise and physical activity.
- List some of the barriers to exercise that may be faced by persons with mental health conditions.
- Suggest some strategies for health promotion.

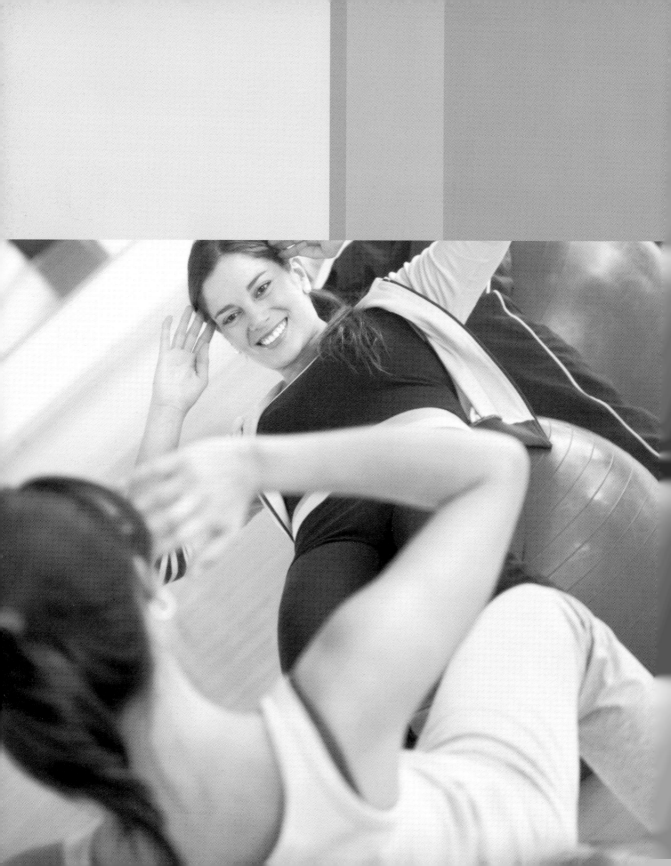

PART TWO

MOTIVATION, BEHAVIOUR CHANGE AND COMMUNICATION

There are many factors that may influence a person's motivation to make changes in different areas of their life. There are equally as many factors that may prevent them from getting started and/ or for continuing or discontinuing with the changes they make.

There have been numerous contributors to the study of motivation, development of personality and behaviour change. This section introduces a few of the psychological models, both old and new, that have proposed various theories to suggest what it is that motivates us and contributes to us becoming the person we are (and the behaviours we choose), or which provides the barriers that cause us to remain stuck in some behaviours. Each theoretical model provides a framework for looking at the subject matter and offers assumptions, which have been accepted or refuted by other theorists. The research into this subject matter is still very much ongoing.

Some strategies for working with clients and communication skills are also introduced as a starting point for continued learning, which needs to be ongoing via reflective practice.

'Clients with mental health issues are the group with the highest number of non-attendances for their first initial consultation. The people that attend from organisations like ARC (Assisted Recovery in the Community) day care centre do tend to turn up for their appointments as ARC usually provides support (a training buddy/carer) to attend with the person during the first couple of weeks. It can be quite difficult for some clients to overcome the barriers that prevent them from joining in, like a busy gym environment/reception – those sorts of issues. On the other hand you can be really surprised by some individuals, who you think will never continue coming and they do! Unfortunately, these people are still a small minority.'

– Stuart Mitchell, Exercise Referral Coordinator, Bridgend Recreation Centre, Wales

// MOTIVATION

4

DEFINITION

The word 'motivation' originates from the Latin word motive, which means 'to move'.

> **Definition**
>
> *Motive:* 'A cause which energises, directs and sustains a person's behaviour'
> – Rubin & McNeil, 1983 in Gross, 1996:9
>
> 'The study of motivation is: "The study of all those pushes and prods – biological, social and psychological – that defeat our laziness and move us, either eagerly or reluctantly, to action"'
> – Miller, 1962 in Gross, 1996:96

Clearly, our 'motives' and our motivation will affect our behaviour and the lifestyle choices we make.

OBJECTIVES

By the end of this chapter, you should be able to:

- recognise different models of motivation and development;
- discuss the client-centred approach and core conditions; and

- recognise self-determination theory as a modern approach/model.

THEORIES OF MOTIVATION

There have been numerous theories and contributors to the study of motivation. The central themes for early philosophers and for humanistic and cognitive theorists are the concepts of freedom and responsibility. This would include the freedom and responsibility that may govern our specific life choices. Refer to Figure 4.1.

PSYCHODYNAMIC THEORIES

Psychodynamic theorists (such as Freud) believed that human beings were driven by **motives** that were unconscious and out of their awareness. These include the drive for both pleasure (Eros) and self-destruction (Thanos). Freud believed that the person we 'see' represented only the tip of an iceberg and the richness in finding the human self was found through uncovering his/her unconscious motives and drives. Psychodynamic theorists believe that the way to reach the unconscious was through the process of analysing dreams and fantasies and through techniques such as 'free association'.

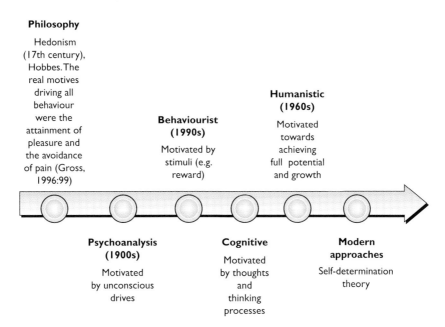

Philosophy

Hedonism (17th century), Hobbes. The real motives driving all behaviour were the attainment of pleasure and the avoidance of pain (Gross, 1996:99)

Behaviourist (1990s)

Motivated by stimuli (e.g. reward)

Humanistic (1960s)

Motivated towards achieving full potential and growth

Psychoanalysis (1900s)

Motivated by unconscious drives

Cognitive

Motivated by thoughts and thinking processes

Modern approaches

Self-determination theory

Figure 4.1 The development of theories of motivation over time

This approach is considered by later theorists as pessimistic, because it views human beings as not having any control or power over their own destiny. The approach has also been refuted by some as it is not possible to provide a scientific evidence base to measure that which is **unconscious**, it cannot be measured directly.

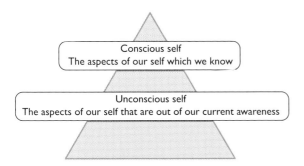

Conscious self
The aspects of our self which we know

Unconscious self
The aspects of our self that are out of our current awareness

Figure 4.2 'Iceberg' representing the conscious and unconscious

Erikson's psychosocial theory of lifespan development

Erikson suggested that to function successfully, specific life lessons need to be accomplished at different stages of life (see Table 4.1). If these lessons were not learned, the person would become stuck in patterns of behaviour, relating to that earlier stage of development. Erikson proposed that unresolved conflicts at each stage (being stuck) may contribute to some of the social problems present in society (e.g. taking drugs and suicide may link to the adolescent stage) and what he referred to as the 'identity crisis' stage.

The model potentially offers the opportunity for stages and lessons to be revisited and relearned at a later stage in life (e.g. through therapy). However, there also exists the possibility for learning to be shattered or shaken 'if later deprivation is experienced,' (Gross, 1996:413).

Table 4.1	Erikson's lifespan development		
Age	Life lesson, crisis or conflict	Significant relationship	Possible learning outcome
0–1	Trust vs. mistrust	Mother figure	Trust and faith or a mistrust of people
1–3	Autonomy vs. shame and doubt	Parents	Self-control and mastery or self-doubt and fearfulness
3–5	Initiative vs. guilt	Family	Purpose and direction or loss of self-esteem
6–11	Industry vs. inferiority	Neighbourhood and school	Competence in social and intellectual pursuits or failure to thrive and develop
Adolescence	Identity vs. role confusion	Peer groups, out-group, models of leadership	Sense of self or uncertainty about one's role in life
Early adulthood	Intimacy vs. isolation	Partners in friendship, sex competition, cooperation	Formation of deep personal relationships or the failure to love others
Middle age	Generativity vs. stagnation	Divided labour and shared household	Expansion of interests and caring for others or inward turning toward one's own problems
Old age	Integrity vs. despair	Human kind, 'my 'kind'	Satisfaction with the triumphs and disappointments of life or a sense of unfulfilment and a fear of death

Erikson's theory has also been criticised, in that the observations were limited to a specific population (middle class white men), which is not representative of other groups, such as women and people from different racial groups (Gross, 1996:413).

HUMANISTIC THEORIES

Humanistic theorists (Rogers & Maslow) take a more positive view of human beings (see Figure 4.3). They state that in the right environment, we are able to be masters of our own destiny.

Person-centred approach (Carl Rogers)

The person-centred approach evolves from the work of Carl Rogers (1967:90) who believed that the 'person is the best expert on themselves'. He proposed that people are capable of working out their own solutions to their problems in the right environment. Rogers believed that motivation and behaviour were a response, by the individual, that related to their perception and interpretation of external stimuli. He believed that: 'Many adult adjustment problems are bound up by attempts to live by other people's standards rather than one's own' (Gross, 1996:764).

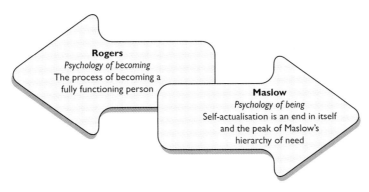

Figure 4.3 Humanistic theorists (adapted from Gross, 1996:763)

The core conditions

The right environment, according to Rogers, was one where the core conditions were present. Rogers believed that if these conditions were present, they enable the person to grow, develop and reach their full potential and become their real self – a self without masks. Alternatively, an environment where these conditions were not fully present would lead us to behave in ways that were not true to our own heart, creating inner conflicts and blocks to our growth.

The role of the helper, for this model, is to facilitate an environment that encourages the person to become the expert on themselves by placing them at the centre of the helping process. This differs from other approaches where the professional person is seen as the 'expert' and offers solutions, that may or may not fit with the 'person' being helped.

The three primary core conditions for building a positive relationship to bring about successful change are:

1   Congruence
2   Empathy
3   Unconditional positive regard

1. Congruence

Rogers suggested that congruence (being true to one's self and own values) and self-actualisation (achieving one's full potential) are enhanced by substituting conditions of worth (where you are valued for something you give or do, rather than for just being who you are) with organismic values (allowing yourself to 'be' who you are and being true to the values of your own heart).

In a helping relationship, congruence is modelled on being totally honest and genuine. The helper presents their whole self, without putting on a front or a façade/mask and encourages the person do the same. This enables the individual to get in touch with their own authentic feelings and thoughts, rather than denying these aspects of self. Positive self-regard is no longer dependent on conditions of worth (Gross, 1996:764). The person is valued, 'warts and all', and learns to value themselves.

To be congruent, the helper needs to be aware of their own thoughts and feelings (this includes prejudices). They need to be able to 'be' with, and manage their own feelings and thoughts, without denying or discounting them. Through this awareness, they may choose to communicate their thoughts or feelings, if and when appropriate.

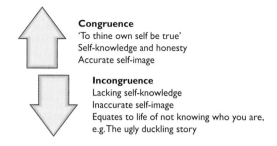

Congruence
'To thine own self be true'
Self-knowledge and honesty
Accurate self-image

Incongruence
Lacking self-knowledge
Inaccurate self-image
Equates to life of not knowing who you are,
e.g. The ugly duckling story

Figure 4.4 Congruence or incongruence

However, congruence should not be confused with the need to 'blurt out impulsively every feeling and accusation under the comfortable impression that one is being genuine' (Rogers, 1967:91) as this is not helpful! Moreover, it is being aware of one's own inner responses and having the resources to process these in a safe environment, enabling the helper the opportunity to continue to learn more about their own self as well. Therapists and counsellors would take these issues and work with them in their supervision.

Most people are able to sense incongruence, when a person is putting on a front to perform a role. People can also recognise when a person is not communicating the things they think or feel and thus, will often hold back from revealing themselves at any deeper level. Alternatively, with a person who is authentic, people are more likely to develop trust and as a consequence be more of who they are.

An essential aspect of congruence is learning to communicate effectively. We communicate messages to others not only with the words we use (7 per cent), but also through our intonation (38 per cent) and body language (55 per cent) – see Figure 6.3 on page 132. Clearly, any discrepancy between what we say and how we feel will be communicated at some level. The response we get from our communication may actually tell us more about what we are communicating than what we say, or how we say it.

2. Empathy

This is the ability to see things from the other person's perspective, to put yourself into their position and understand their world as if it were your own, without losing the 'as if' quality (Rogers, 1967:93). In order to do this we need to be aware of any prejudices and closed-mindedness (personal congruence) within us and put these issues to one side. We also need to be able to put to one side any need to analyse and evaluate, which only serves to see the person's world from our own perspective. It does not lead to us understanding theirs.

Removing the barriers to intimacy (judgement, prejudice and ignorance) will help to minimise projection of our own issues into the other person's world. It will also help us to know the other person, from their perspective. Our communication skills are once again of key importance. Appropriate questioning and inquiry enable the person to tell their own story and the helper can use reflective statements and paraphrasing to mirror their empathy.

Empathy is powerful, as Rogers (1967:93) quotes: 'When someone understands how it feels and seems to be me, without wanting to analyse me or judge me, then I can blossom and grow in that climate'.

3. Unconditional positive regard

Unconditional positive regard is about **acceptance** and showing respect and warmth for the person (see Figure 4.5). It is about prizing them as an individual in their own right, valuing the way they manage their struggles, appreciating their own unique way of being and valuing who they are without making judgements or decisions that they should be any other way.

It is fairly normal for human beings to dislike and judge certain human behaviours and have prejudices. However, in order to demonstrate unconditional positive regard one needs to be aware of these and take responsibility for processing these judgements as a growing aspect of self. These judgements should not be used to condemn or disempower another person.

For example, working with a client who frequently lapses from their activity plan may stir up feelings of frustration or disappointment inside, which may raise judgements inside the helper (they are lazy, unmotivated, etc.). The feelings need to be acknowledged internally within the helper as an aspect of themselves (personal congruence).

To develop empathy, the helper can ask the person how they feel about the lapse. This enables them to use their own voice and describe their own feelings in response to the situation, which gives a truer picture of their world as they see it and experience it (it may be that they also feel frustrated and disappointed). The process can be moved forward by asking them: 'How can we work together to move through this barrier?'

Building an open channel for communication can provide the helper with an opportunity to highlight that these feelings are a natural response to lapses. They can also point out that further self-berating (which often occurs after a lapse) and judgement are not helpful. The person may learn to recognise their own inner judge – the aspect of self that likes to criticise and focus on the negative; and the inner nurturer – the aspect of self that is able pick us up, dust us down and help us move forward and see the positive steps we make (Stewart & Joines,1987). Strengthening the nurturing aspect of the person can help them to help themselves and become their own best friend. This nurturing (self-valuing) aspect of self can also help the person to balance any inner conflicts they may experience.

Unconditional positive regard
An environment providing love and acceptance for the whole person ('warts and all') enables the person to operate in a way that is true to their organismic self, which enables growth

Conditional positive regard
An environment where love, acceptance and approval are withheld unless behaviour conform to the 'norms' stifles growth,
e.g. Learning to behave in specific ways to gain approval and acceptance (from parents and society), rather than behaving in a way that is more intrinsically satisfying and real/authentic (which may include, displaying anger or fear or grief)

Conditions of worth become internalised and reflect on the way we see ourselves, e.g. To be loved, accepted, approved of I must be perfect, work hard, not show my feelings, be good, etc.

Figure 4.5 Unconditional vs. conditional positive regard

Table 4.2	Person- and non-person-centred approach (adapted from Waine, 2002)
Person-centred approach	**Non-person-centred approach**
Being empathic	Being unconcerned about the person's struggles in relation to their condition
Being unbiased	Being judgemental about the person, which includes being aware of any pre-judgements, self-righteousness and blame regarding the person's contribution and responsibility for their condition from their behaviour choices (inactivity, smoking, alcohol misuse, poor eating habits, risk-taking behaviours, self-harm, etc.)
Being supportive	Being dismissive
Being accepting	Fault finding and blaming
Being optimistic	Being sceptical
Highlighting the positive changes that can be made by simple and achievable adjustments and the positive impact that each small change can make	

From a helper's perspective, lapses and relapses can be viewed as acknowledgement that the approach selected was not of 'best fit' for the person at that point in time. Lapses offer the potential to learn more about the person and enables exploration of other ways of making changes.

As exercise professionals, we need to recognise that while we may have certain pieces of knowledge that may be helpful to the person we are working with, it is the client who knows their lifestyle and what changes will work for them in their life and they have the freedom and responsibility to make their own choices. If a person resists our 'useful' suggestions we can acknowledge that somehow this is not right for this person. A more effective approach is to ask the person what they really want and explore a range of potential ways to help them reach their goal.

Person-centred working does not necessarily provide the 'quick fix', if indeed there is such a thing. However, it is a way of working that enables effective change in the longer term.

Self-actualisation (Abraham Maslow)

Maslow believed that the human tendency was to grow towards self-actualisation, but that blocks to the fulfilment of specific needs would hinder that growth.

On the hierarchy (see Figure 4.6), the lower needs (deficiency needs) are the priority and once fulfilled, this allows movement towards the growth needs. The deficiency needs are a means to an end, the growth needs are an end in themselves.

Exclusion is a barrier to growth. We all need to feel like we belong (inclusion) and are loved (a deficiency need) to grow towards our full potential. There is so much stigma around the area of mental health that people with mental health conditions may feel excluded. They may try to dismiss or disguise their condition and keep it a personal

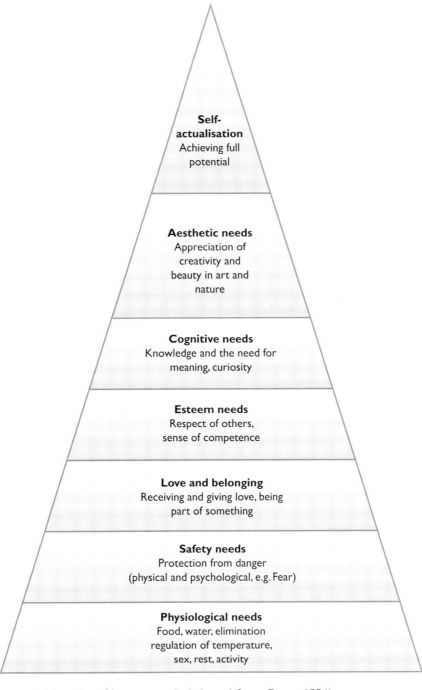

Figure 4.6 Maslow's hierarchy of human needs (adapted from Gross, 1996)

secret, for fear of being judged and not accepted. This secret is an incongruence for the person and can prevent them from relating authentically. It can also prevent some people from asking for help and support from family, friends and at work.

Self-determination theory (SDT)

SDT was introduced in 1995 by Richard Ryan and Edward Deci from the University of Rochester in New York. They suggest that human beings can either be proactive and engaged or passive and alienated, and that this is largely in response to the social conditions in which the person develops and functions (see Figure 4.7).

The territory of self-determination theory is the interrelationship between intrinsic and extrinsic motivation and our innate human needs (see Figure 4.8).

The model maintains that people are motivated by their **innate needs** for competence, autonomy and relatedness (see Figure 4.9).

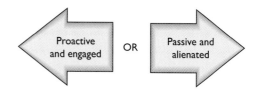

Figure 4.7 Self-determination theory (SDT) showing a continuum of motivation

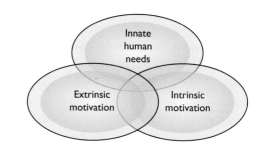

Figure 4.8 The territory of self-determination theory

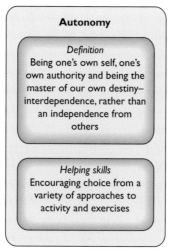
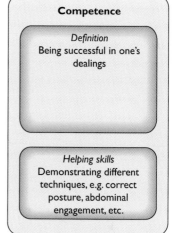

Relatedness	Autonomy	Competence
Definition Being connected to others and experiencing care	*Definition* Being one's own self, one's own authority and being the master of our own destiny—interdependence, rather than an independence from others	*Definition* Being successful in one's dealings
Helping skills Listening to and acknowledging the client's concerns (empathy)	*Helping skills* Encouraging choice from a variety of approaches to activity and exercises	*Helping skills* Demonstrating different techniques, e.g. correct posture, abdominal engagement, etc.

Figure 4.9 Innate human needs

SDT is an integrative model, with humanistic, positivist and person-centred core values. It starts with the basic assumption that people are active organisms and have an evolved tendency towards growth, and that mastery of challenges and the integration of new experiences enable the development of a coherent sense of self. A further assumption is that these aspects of self need to be nourished socially for the individual to flourish (see www.psych.rochester.edu/SDT/theory.php). Alternatively, in an environment where these basic needs are blocked or unnourished, the darker sides of human behaviour and experience (psychopathology, prejudice and aggression) may present.

SDT researchers have explored the effects of a **controlling/didactic environment**, as opposed to an **autonomous and supportive** environment, and how these influence functioning and wellness. SDT theorists follow the humanistic tradition in that they maintain the view that individuals are competent beings, who are able to make the right choices for themselves, and this is paramount to their engagement and ultimate success.

As an integrative model, SDT considers five other specific theories, which contribute ideas to their study of motivation (see Figure 4.10).

1. Cognitive evaluation theory (CET)

Focuses on **intrinsic motivation** – the motivation to behave or do something 'for its own sake'. CET highlights the role of competence and autonomy in fostering intrinsic motivation.

2. Organismic integration theory (OIT)

OIT focuses on **extrinsic motivation** and the extent to which it is internalised. The subtypes of extrinsic motivation, which are seen as falling along a continuum towards **internalisation**, include: External regulation, introjection, identification and integration.

OIT suggests that the 'More internalised the extrinsic motivation the more autonomous the person will be'. OIT highlights the importance of autonomy and relatedness as critical to internalisation. The theory also explores the social contexts that enhance or delay internalisation – that is, the factors that will affect whether the person resists, partially adopts or deeply internalises specific values, goals or beliefs (Ryan and Deci, 1995).

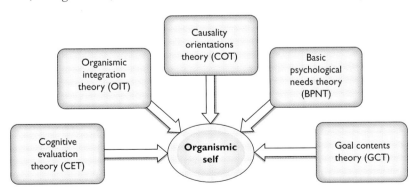

Figure 4.10 Sub-theories of SDT

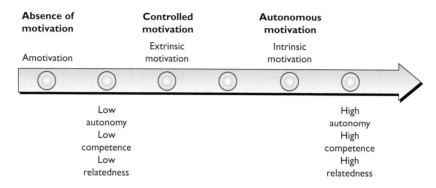

Figure 4.11 Motivation continuum (adapted from www.youtube.com/watch?v=6N_RFNfMjg4)

3. Causality orientations theory (COT)

COT describes the individual differences to orientate toward **environments** and regulate behaviour. COT describes and assesses three types of orientation:

1 The autonomy orientation in which persons act out of interest in and valuing of what is occurring
2 The control orientation in which the focus is on rewards, gains and approval
3 Impersonal or amotivated orientation characterised by anxiety concerning competence.

4. Basic psychological needs theory (BPNT)

BPNT argues that psychological well-being and optimal functioning is predicated on autonomy, competence and relatedness. Contexts that support these needs should invariantly influence wellness; BPNT looks at cross-developmental and cross-cultural settings for validation and refinements.

5. Goal contents theory (GCT)

GCT studies have attempted to make a distinction between intrinsic and extrinsic goals that satisfy specific basic needs and the extent to which these affect our motivation and well-being (see Figure 4.12). The research suggests that intrinsic goals are those that foster higher levels of well-being and motivation.

Key points

• Conditions supporting **autonomy**, **competence** and **relatedness** will foster greater motivation and engagement.
• Motivation that is based on the satisfactions of behaving 'for its own sake'. Doing something because you want to do it.
• The more internalised the extrinsic motivation the more autonomous the person.
• Intrinsic goals are those that foster higher levels of well-being and motivation (see Figure 4.11).

SDT addresses the central questions: Why do people do what they do, and also what are the costs and benefits of various ways of socially regulating or promoting specific behaviours?

Extrinsic motivation	Intrinsic motivation

• Associated with lower wellness and well-being, e.g.
  • Fame and fortune
  • Financial success
  • Appearance
	• Associated with higher wellness and well-being, e.g.
	  • Relationships, love and belonging
	  • Community
	  • Close relationships
	  • Personal development and growth

Figure 4.12 Intrinsic and extrinsic motivation

SDT research and mindfulness

SDT researchers have more recently begun to explore the concept of mindfulness and its relationship with autonomous functioning and emotional well-being. Mindfulness is being fully present in the moment and paying attention to self and environment. It has connections with emotional intelligence that links with good social skills, greater empathy and a willingness to cooperate. Being mindful means we are less likely to 'react' (aggressively or passively) and instead 'respond' to our environment. Being mindful also reduces addictive behaviour and helps us to resist the need to act on impulse.

SDT studies have concluded that when individuals act mindfully, their actions are consistent with their values and interest. They also posit the possibility that being autonomous and performing something because it is enjoyable increases mindful attention to actions.

The practice of mindfulness has gained more attention recently and is being promoted as a method for helping people cope and manage depression and stress. Resilience is built up by teaching people to look out for the warning signs, spot them and deal with them with kindness and compassion rather than harshness, criticism or judgement. Some of the benefits include:

- More able to override or change inner thoughts and feelings
- Less neurotic
- Less risk of depression and anxiety
- More extroverted
- Greater well-being and life satisfaction
- Greater awareness, understanding and acceptance of emotions
- More stable self-esteem, less dependent on external factors
- Better communication
- Improved relationships

Mindfulness involves integration and connection of the reasonable rational and logical mind with the emotional mind (that which deals with feelings) (see Figure 4.13).

SDT research and exercise

SDT research indicates that the more supportive the environment, the more positive the impact on self-determined motivation. An environment where peers are supportive and where there is an emphasis on cooperation, effort and personal improvement (a sense of community), will influence other variables such as basic psychological needs, motivation and enjoyment.

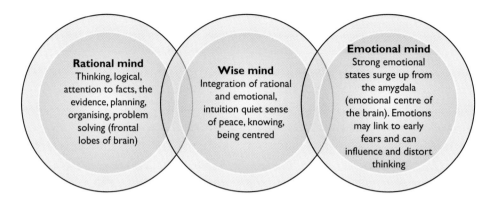

Figure 4.13 Mindfulness and integration

SDT offers a broad framework for the study of motivation and personality. Theorists suggest that conditions which support an individual's experience of **autonomy**, **competence** and **relatedness** are those that will foster the most volitional and quality forms of motivation and engagement, whereas, conditions where these experiences are blocked will have a detrimental impact on wellness in that setting.

SDT research continues to evolve and has been applied to a number of different areas (education, relationships, nutrition, organisations, physical activity, psychotherapy and many others).

Locus of control theory

One major type of competence motive is the need to be in control of our own destiny (Gross, 1996: 113). If freedom is threatened, the reaction is to reassert this (psychological reactance). If loss of control is repeatedly experienced, this may develop learned helplessness (Seligman, 1975 in Gross, 1996:117).

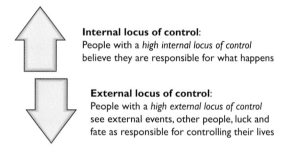

Internal locus of control:
People with a *high internal locus of control* believe they are responsible for what happens

External locus of control:
People with a *high external locus of control* see external events, other people, luck and fate as responsible for controlling their lives

Figure 4.14 Locus of control theory

Cognitive consistency and the need for achievement are two important motives. These are related to features of self-efficacy theory – the fear of failure or possibly the fear of success. The key is to find out whether people have stronger internal or external locus and then persuade them accordingly (see Figure 4.14 and the self-efficacy theory, page 116). For an individual with a higher internal locus, you might show how they are in control and let them choose behaviours. For an individual with a higher external locus of control, you might choose to show how they are being driven by external forces and then offer a middle ground, which may represent a safe haven and starting point for them.

As a starting point, a helper may need to become aware of their own locus of control as this may impact how they work with others. Figure 4.15 shows some questions that will help you check your own locus of control.

SUMMARY POINTS

You should now be able to:

- Recognise different models of motivation.
- Discuss the client-centred approach and core conditions.
- Recognise different models of behaviour change.
- Describe some of the interventions to help a client move through different stages of the change process.

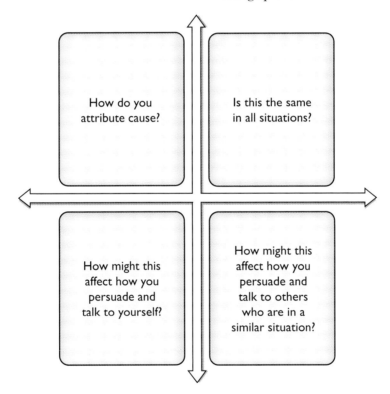

Figure 4.15 Checking your own locus of control

BEHAVIOUR CHANGE

5

Supporting clients who would like to change specific behaviours requires an understanding of motivation and theories of behaviour change. There have been numerous contributors to this field of research. Some models proposed have included: The health belief model; the exercise behaviour model; the theory of reasoned action and the theory of planned behaviour. Each of these have offered valuable contributions to the subject of behaviour change. The approaches discussed in this chapter include:

- Self-efficacy theory
- The trans-theoretical model
- The health action process approach (HAPA)

OBJECTIVES

By the end of this chapter you should be able to:

- recognise different models of behaviour change; and
- recognise strategies suggested by each model to assist clients with changing behaviour.

SELF-EFFICACY THEORY (ALBERT BANDURA)

Self-efficacy theory evolved from the work of Albert Bandura (1977) whose studies focused on how thinking processes may influence behaviour change (cognitive behaviour modification). Self-efficacy focuses on an individual's **perceived confidence** regarding their ability to perform a specific action or behaviour or task, for example:

- confidence to start an exercise programme;
- confidence to stop smoking;
- confidence to attend a study group; and/or
- confidence to perform a cartwheel.

Wise words

'Whether you think you can, whether you think you cannot, you are 100 per cent correct!'

– Henry Ford

Bandura believed that an individual's perception of their ability was a key factor in determining their motivation:

- to initiate a change (intention);
- to expend effort while making the change (volition); and
- to persist and keep going (adherence).

For example, an individual who perceived they *could* do something (change a behaviour or perform a task) would be more inclined to take on the challenge and keep it going; whereas an individual who *did not* believe they could do something would be less likely to start the task, and if they did, would be less likely to keep it going (relapse).

Bandura also believed that there were two key aspects of efficacy that would influence confidence in exercise and physical activity:

1 **Efficacy expectations:** An individual's beliefs about their own self-competence
2 **Outcome expectations:** An individual's beliefs regarding the perceived result or outcome of doing something. For example, if a person believes that something will not work, then it is likely that it will not.

Bandura (1977) identified four primary sources that inform self-efficacy:

1 **Performance attainment:** Possibly the most powerful of the four, because it is based on personal experience of success or failure. Success increases efficacy, whereas, failure reduces it. Failure may be linked to previous negative experiences, especially those that are attached to a negative emotion being evoked, such as humiliation or shame, e.g. coming last in a race at school, or being the one always picked last for a team or being consciously aware that you are the only one in an exercise class who is not able to keep up.

2 **Imitation and modelling:** Seeing others who are very similar to yourself succeed or fail can enhance one's own self-efficacy if they have no prior experience. For example, seeing a person with the same mental health condition taking part in exercise or completing the marathon can create the feeling 'if they can do it, so can I' – the expert patient programme offers the potential for this. The expert patient programme asks service users to share their experiences with other new people, going through the same problem – this can be mental health or physical health, e.g. recovering from heart surgery. Alternatively, having a role model (an elite athlete or sporting star) can provide a motivational goal – 'I want to be like that'.

3 **Verbal and social persuasion:** Being influenced by another person to do something, which may be effective, if the person's opinion is respected and valued.

4 **Judgements of physical states:** How the person interprets a physiological response. This is of particular relevance for people with mental health conditions as many of the initial physiological effects of exercise (increased heart rate, sweating, increased breathlessness,

etc.) are the same as the side effects of some medication and as the symptoms of some mental conditions (e.g. panic attacks).

RE-STRUCTURING STRATEGIES

You can support change by enabling the **restructuring** of an individual's thinking (cognitive) processes and help them to reframe any negative perceptions and experiences they may have, especially with regard to physical activity and exercise. Some re-structuring strategies include:

- Providing education regarding the immediate effects of exercise (e.g. 'you will start to feel warm and your heart rate may increase and you may begin to perspire,' etc.) may help an individual to recognise their body's response to the exercise, rather than it being a symptom of a condition or a response to their medication.
- Providing a positive environment where individuals are valued and supported (core conditions).
- Offering adaptations and alternatives to promote inclusion, rather than creating exclusion.
- Offering praise, especially to newcomers who may need assistance in building their confidence.
- Promoting exercise as a reward, rather than a punishment! For example, encouraging exercise as a daily reward for the self (taking care of themselves), rather than promoting it as a compensatory behaviour for eating too much (a punishment).
- Promoting self-monitoring rather than competition.
- Promoting the use of positive self-talk, which the person can use to assist their efficacy and motivation before and during exercise.

- Providing resources (handouts, fact sheets, etc.) that give information on the positive effects of exercise.
- Promoting the rewards of exercise (health and other benefits).
- Being mindful of the individual's physiological response that occurs when they think about exercising, e.g. 'this is boring' or 'I don't like it' etc. This may be out of their conscious awareness, but has the potential to be a large barrier to participation. For example, if an individual inwardly groans at the thought of exercise and perceives exercise as hard work or a punishment, then this cognition will need to be reframed.

THE TRANS-THEORETICAL MODEL OF CHANGE

The trans-theoretical model describes a 'staged' approach of readiness to change and is based on the premise that trying to push a person to change something before they are ready will hit a wall of resistance and/or may trigger premature lapse (a temporary slip up) or relapse (return to an old behaviour).

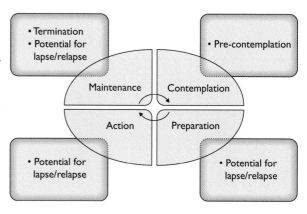

Figure 5.1 Stages of behaviour change

Table 5.1   Stages and interventions

Stage and attitude	Aim	Intervention
Pre-contemplation: • Resistant to change • Feelings of powerlessness and helplessness • Fear of changing or denial of problem	Provide information that may assist the person to move closer towards contemplating making a change	• Handouts • Leaflets • Person-centred interviewing to explore resistance
Contemplation: • Considering making changes to behaviour • Internal conflicts regarding decision to change • Can become stuck at this stage unless specific interventions	Explore the advantages and disadvantages of both changing and not changing and also explore the risk and harm caused by their existing behaviour	• Decisional balance • Behaviour recording diaries
Preparation: • Ready to change • Small changes made	Keep on track	• SMART (specific, measurable, achievable, realistic and relevant, time framed) targets • Motivation • Rewards • Coping strategies
Action: • Changes made (one day to six months)	Keeping motivated	• Coping strategies for stimulus control, e.g. alternative behaviours to triggers
Maintenance: • Changes sustained beyond six months • Some coping strategies in place	Sustaining the change and preventing relapse	• Helpful and supportive relationship • Reinforce positive behaviour • Praise and encouragement and reward • Increase self-efficacy • Remind of successes • Raise awareness of cues for likelihood of relapse • Teach coping strategies
Relapse or lapse: • Returned to their old behaviour • Momentary slip up from new behaviour	Get back on track	• Support and encouragement • Explore possible causes for the relapse • Review and create action plan
Termination	Permanent change achieved	

STAGES AND SUGGESTED INTERVENTIONS

In reality, the process shown in table 5.1 is not so orderly; people get stuck at specific stages and lapse or relapse and enter the cycle a few times before they move towards permanent changes.

The model may help to identify the different levels of psychological functioning (see Figure 5.2) which interrelate and which require work to help the person make the desired changes.

Recognising where the person is within the cycle of change enables the helper to identify the appropriate interventions for which they are qualified to manage, and those where their expertise ends and additional professional support, such as counselling or other intervention, is required.

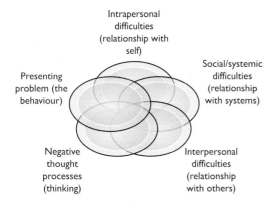

Figure 5.2 Different levels of psychological functioning

AWARENESS-RAISING TO ASSIST WITH CHANGE

Prochaska and Diclemente (1984) name 10 common processes that people involved in a changing and growth process move through (Feltham, 2000:400).

1   **Consciousness-raising and self-monitoring:** These are methods for gathering information about oneself and the problem(s) and monitoring and raising awareness to triggers to specific lifestyle choices. They include the use of diaries and a list of all the things that 'hassle' you.

2   **Self-liberation:** Taking a positive approach and believing in the possibility of change and making the choice to commit to take action.

3   **Social liberation:** Raising awareness of the increasing opportunity for alternative behaviours in society, e.g. active transport (walking, cycling, etc.).

4   **Counter-conditioning:** Introducing alternative behaviour to the specific problem behaviour. For example, when stress is triggered, taking a few deep breaths, rather than just reacting.

5   **Stimulus control:** Using specific techniques to reduce the stimuli that trigger specific behaviours, e.g. not visiting specific environments.

6   **Self-reevaluation:** Evaluating how one thinks and feels about their self in relation to the problem behaviour or medical condition. The stigma attached to mental health may be **internalised** within some people with mental health conditions and this may need to be worked on with the support of a counsellor.

7   **Environmental reevaluation:** Recognising how the problem behaviour affects the family, relatives, the broader physical community and environment, for example, a person who is abusing alcohol or drugs will need to be aware of the impact of their behaviour.

8   **Contingency/reinforcement management:** These techniques involve giving the self a

reward or a creature comfort when a single small change has been made. Rewards can include:

- Small rewards (a bubble bath, watching a favourite video, etc.)
- Medium rewards (buying a new outfit, a body massage, etc.)
- Larger rewards (a holiday or health spa retreat, etc.)

9 **Dramatic relief:** Experiencing and expressing feelings that may be linked with the problem behaviour and identifying possible solutions to manage these. For example, there are support groups where people with addictive behaviours or eating disorders can express the feelings that may be holding them in a negative behaviour cycle.

10 **Helping relationships and support systems:** Receiving appropriate support and encouragement is a key factor to assisting with the management of behaviour change. It is essential to have a support system of people who care and who the person is able to trust to speak openly to about the problems they may be experiencing. Some people struggle with asking for help and support and others struggle with finding the support they need. This is especially true for people with mental health conditions because of the stigma that surrounds mental health. Other blocks that prevent a person from social interaction and support can include: Low self-esteem, self-belief, low assertiveness, depression, habitually doing things alone, etc. Clients need to be encouraged to build a support system proactively (calling friends, joining groups, etc.) and decreasing the number of activities they take part in alone.

MOTIVATIONAL INTERVIEWING

Motivational interviewing is a client-centred method of gathering information to explore a client's readiness to change. It can be used to elicit information about the client's concerns about specific areas of their life that they would like to change. This information can be then be used to discuss with the person the advantages and disadvantages of making changes they propose. The information collected can also indicate where the client is in relation to the cycle-of-change model (contemplating, preparing and acting) (see Figure 5.1) and can identify their personal levels of motivation and the support systems they have in place. It can also help to identify any resistance or ambivalence the person has to making changes. All of this information aids the exercise professional in providing the appropriate support and intervention to help the client make a positive decision for themselves. Finally, it enables the exercise professional to negotiate goals and strategies to work towards with their client.

10-STEP APPROACH

The 10-step approach can be used to assist people to manage their own change process (see Figure 5.3).

HEALTH ACTION PROCESS APPROACH (HAPA)

HAPA suggests that changing behaviour is a process that consists of two main phases (see Figure 5.4):

1 The motivation phase (setting the intention, deciding to make a change)
2 The volition phase (following the intention through to action; the steps to making the change happen – planning, action, maintenance)

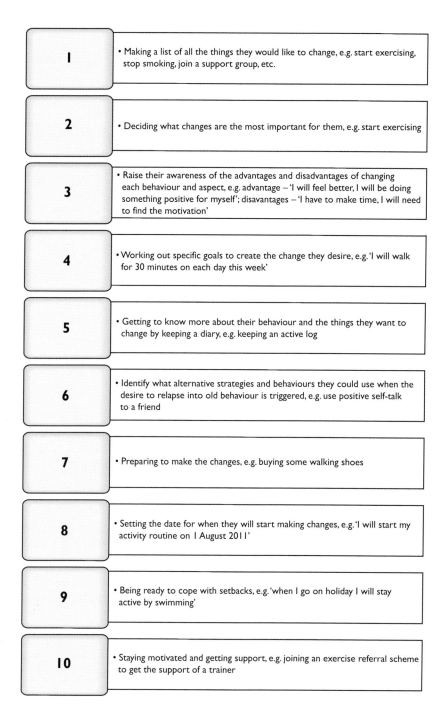

Figure 5.3 The 10-step approach

1 • Making a list of all the things they would like to change, e.g. start exercising, stop smoking, join a support group, etc.

2 • Deciding what changes are the most important for them, e.g. start exercising

3 • Raise their awareness of the advantages and disadvantages of changing each behaviour and aspect, e.g. advantage – 'I will feel better, I will be doing something positive for myself'; disavantages – 'I have to make time, I will need to find the motivation'

4 • Working out specific goals to create the change they desire, e.g. 'I will walk for 30 minutes on each day this week'

5 • Getting to know more about their behaviour and the things they want to change by keeping a diary, e.g. keeping an active log

6 • Identify what alternative strategies and behaviours they could use when the desire to relapse into old behaviour is triggered, e.g. use positive self-talk to a friend

7 • Preparing to make the changes, e.g. buying some walking shoes

8 • Setting the date for when they will start making changes, e.g. 'I will start my activity routine on 1 August 2011'

9 • Being ready to cope with setbacks, e.g. 'when I go on holiday I will stay active by swimming'

10 • Staying motivated and getting support, e.g. joining an exercise referral scheme to get the support of a trainer

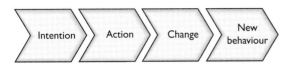

Figure 5.4 The HAPA model viewed as a continuum

Success at each stage and throughout the process can be predicted by one's self-efficacy. Quite simply, the more a person believes they are capable of making a change, the higher the likelihood for success. On the other hand, any self-doubt and lack of self-belief will make it less likely that a change will be initiated, let alone maintained.

Other processes

Other thinking processes that are influential at the motivational stage, when the person is contemplating making changes include:

- **Outcome expectancies:** The result/outcome we anticipate
- **Risk perceptions:** The risk we attach to maintaining a specific behaviour (e.g. the risk of inactivity, smoking, etc.) as opposed to changing

The motivation phase

This is the phase where the individual forms an intention to make a change. The intended change may be either adopting a precautionary measure or changing a high risk or negative behaviour to another healthier behaviour.

The major predictors from which intentions manifest are **self-efficacy** and **outcome expectancy**, that is, one's self-belief to undertake the necessary actions to make the change happen and the anticipated result (consequences) of

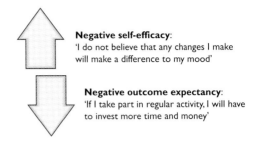

Figure 5.5 Lower volition

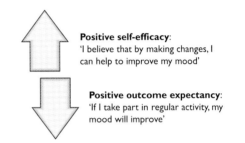

Figure 5.6 Higher volition

making the change. The more positive the self-belief, and the more positive the anticipated outcome, the higher the likelihood will be to put the intention into action.

Most people will weigh up the consequences (their expected or anticipated outcome) of doing something before they question their potential competence and ability to succeed and achieve. This is even more likely in circumstances where the person has no experience of the contemplated behaviour change. For example, one positive **expected outcome** for quitting smoking could be the money the person will save. A person who has never attempted to give up smoking will not have any experience of changing that behaviour, thus their intention would be more motivated by the expected outcome (saving money, an external motivator), than their self-efficacy (ability to achieve their goal, an internal motivator), so they may be motivated to 'have a go' and may well succeed. Alternatively, a person who has tried to give up smoking in the past and relapsed may well find that their self-talk and perceived efficacy (which is low, because they have 'failed' before) diffuses the formation of any further positive intentions (they give up before they have even started), despite the attractiveness of the expected outcome.

A further predictor is **risk perception**. While a minimum level of threat needs to be recognised before any change is contemplated, appealing to fear doesn't always work. There have been numerous campaigns to promote the consequences for health of maintaining specific behaviours, such as smoking, drinking, bad diet, inactivity, etc.), yet the problem behaviours continue to persist.

The HAPA model suggests that the message in any persuasive techniques should be framed in a way that allows individuals to identify and draw on their coping resources and their potential ability to exercise skills to control health threats. Rather than emphasising and enlarging the fear, the emphasis is instead placed on the potential competence of the person to cope and manage, the element of fear is minimised and promoted as something they can manage and something they can handle.

The volition phase

This is the phase where intentions become action – our determination and will or how hard we will try and how long we will keep going (and stay on the pathway) to getting where we want to go (intention).

Once an intention has been shaped in the motivation phase, this has to be framed as a detailed set of instructions that provide a guide for to how to get there. For example, a person with the intention to be more active will need specific guidance on how often they need to be active and for how long; what type of activities they need to undertake; what to wear; how this will develop over time, etc. Using the analogy of a pathway the intention is on where the person is going and the instructions are the steps they need to take to get there.

The volitional phase and execution of will is mainly influenced by self-efficacy, which determines both the effort the person puts in and the perseverance to sustain the change (see Figures 5.5 and 5.6). In practice, an individual with a higher self-efficacy (competence and experience) may have a higher number and higher quality (more challenging) of action plans (bigger steps to making the change); whereas, an individual with lower self-efficacy would be encouraged to work towards smaller targets and with fewer action plans initially, with the aim being to build their efficacy. In essence, they would need to take a 'one step at a time' approach to making changes.

Strategies (meta-cognitions) will be needed to maintain efforts and avoid distractions during the volition phase. For example, sticking to a healthy eating plan will need self-regulation to keep up the effort and overcome any cravings to eat unhealthy foods and/or avoid temptation situations (passing the cake shop, take-away meals, etc.) until the new behaviour has been established.

Visualisation

People with a lower self-efficacy may anticipate failure and doubt their ability to handle situations, which may contribute to them prematurely aborting their attempt to make changes.

Alternatively, people with a higher and more positive self-efficacy are more likely to visualise success and find ways of coping and persevering when obstacles arise. They are also more able to recover from relapse scenarios more effectively because they are more able to regain self-control. For example, if they are craving an unhealthy snack, a cigarette or a drink, they are more able to survive the critical situation. The more developed the meta-cognitive processes and the closer they are matched to specific risk situations, the easier the urges will be to manage. What this means is that the person will have the experience of being in the situation before and will be aware that they have the strategies to manage the situation and should therefore survive the potentially will-breaking risk.

However, there are other social and situational barriers that will also impact cognitive control. For example, a person who is quitting smoking and who is able to gain the support of their social network to remain abstinent from smoking in their presence will be more empowered than a smoker who is unable to secure that social support. Being in the latter situations would place an additional stress on their will power.

HAPA AS A STAGE MODEL

Table 5.2	Stages and interventions		
Stage	**Aim**	**Intention**	**Action**
Interventions	Risk and resource communication, e.g. decisional balance, information handouts	Strategic planning, e.g. goal setting, commitment setting	Relapse prevention , e.g. avoidance of high risk situations, awareness of triggers, etc.

Table 5.3	Stages and interventions	
Motivation phase	**Volition phase**	
Intention, e.g. building the pathways to establishing the intention to change	Coping self-efficacy, e.g. setting goals and preparing for setbacks	Recovery/relapse efficacy, e.g. maintaining self-efficacy and engagement in the event of relapse
Perceived self-efficacy, e.g. 'I believe I can do it' or 'I don't believe I can do it'	Action planning	• Action • Initiative • Maintenance • Recovery
Outcome expectancy, e.g. 'I believe I will succeed' or 'I don't believe I will succeed'	Coping strategy planning	• Barriers and resources
Risk perception, e.g. 'I believe I am able to manage risk situations' or 'I am afraid that I will not be able to manage risk situations'	Positive mental attitude: 'I can handle it'	• Disengagement or engagement; off the wagon or on the wagon

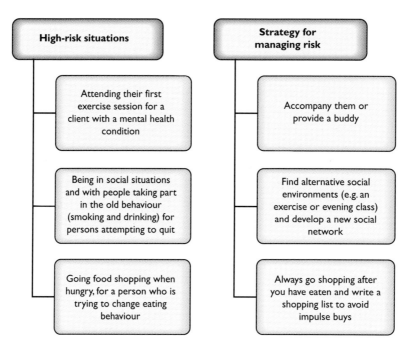

Figure 5.7 Examples of high-risk situations and strategies to avoid a relapse situation

RELAPSE PREVENTION AND MANAGEMENT

Relapse and returning to old behaviours is always a risk for persons involved in changing. The risk of relapse is particularly high for people with mental health conditions, as the symptoms of the condition and affects of medication significantly impact their motivation, mood and behaviour.

A useful first strategy is to identify situations where the person will be most at risk of relapsing. Once the high-risk situation has been identified, strategies can be put in place to either prevent (proactive) or manage (reactive) the situation. See Figure 5.7 for examples of this.

Relapse can destroy the will of those who start with the highest aspirations. It can trigger feelings of failure and push the person to return to their old behaviour, and can leave them feeling incompetent (feeling useless and hopeless). Strategies for promoting adherence and preventing relapse may include:

- Setting **SMART targets** (specific, measurable, achievable/agreed, realistic, time-framed) enables success. There may be an ambitious and broad long-term goal (to give up something such as smoking, or start something (exercise) but the short-term and immediate goals should be more easy and realistic to achieve and planned on a day by day (even minute by minute) basis. For example, 'today I will walk for 15 minutes on the way to and from work'. Goals also need to motivate the person and give them a spark of excitement because if they don't, then the likelihood is that the goal won't be important to them.

- Having a **contingency plan** (ways to stay or get back on the wagon) for any potential or actual setbacks, e.g. phoning a buddy in situations when the temptation to revert to an old behaviour arises). Some referral schemes provide a service where they telephone the client to help motivate them to attend a session.
- Taking one step and one day at a time – for example, eating one cream cake and breaking the diet doesn't mean the diet has failed, it is one slip up at one point in time. We can balance the slip by being sensible for the rest of the day.
- Highlighting the benefits of making change – accentuating the positive. Stay focused on the reasons for making the change.
- Encouraging and developing positive self-talk, rather than self-berating (e.g. 'I can do this, I can handle this' as opposed to 'I will never be able to do this').
- Rewarding success and achievements – making note of every single positive aspect, so that the slip ups and relapses can be seen in a realistic perspective (they are only a small part of an overall more successful attempt to change). Using a notebook to record all the successes of the day that relate the goal, e.g. for someone with depression – 'I got up when my alarm went off and ran and bathed and got dressed'.
- Reframing setbacks – seeing them as a natural part of the process, rather than failure, and keeping them in perspective by highlighting positive achievements as well (e.g. we all slip up, this is natural and part of the process of making changes and it is okay! We can learn from the experience and move on to achieve what we want to achieve).

- Providing support systems – support groups, family and helpful friends (e.g. we need to surround ourselves with people who encourage and support us to make changes).
- Providing positive feedback – everyone needs a positive cheering squad.
- Providing education – when appropriate explain to clients with mental health conditions that the condition and medication will impact motivation. Encourage them to take control, rather than let the condition control them (e.g. when you feel depressed the motivation to do anything physical just leaves the spirit, yet, movement enhances the spirit. It is helpful of the exercise professional is aware of this and can provide the encouragement for the person, when they cannot provide it for themselves).
- Providing access to expert patients – people who live with the condition and maintain positive behaviours. Let them tell and share their story as a way of demonstrating that there is a way forward (e.g. people who have lived the experience and know what it is like can be inspiring – 'if they can do it, so can I'.
- Providing information about other services that can support the person.

SUMMARY POINTS
You should now be able to:

- Recognise different models of behaviour change.
- Describe some of the interventions to help a client move through different stages of the change process.

// COMMUNICATION

6

Effective communication is an art. However, there are specific skills that can be learned through continued practice and reflection. The art is to be open to continued learning.

Communication needs to be adapted to meet the needs of different circumstances and within different settings and with different people. The way we communicate with our family members and friends may be different to the way we communicate at work and with professional colleagues.

This section initially outlines the main stages of the 'working alliance'. It then explores different communication skills and other factors that may influence the effectiveness of our communication.

OBJECTIVES

By the end of this chapter you should be able to:

- recognise the main stages of the working alliance;
- recognise the main communication at each stage of the alliance;
- recognise different communication skills (active listening and questioning);
- appreciate other factors that may influence the effectiveness of communication; and
- differentiate assertive communication from other styles of communication.

THE WORKING ALLIANCE

Establishing and maintaining an effective working alliance and relationship is one of the key factors that will determine the effectiveness of the work. The working alliance and professional relationship contract comprises of three stages (see Figure 6.1).

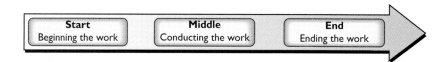

Figure 6.1 The three stages of the working alliance

1. BEGINNING THE WORK

The first meeting with the person/s you are working with can create lasting impressions. This is why it essential to dress and behave appropriately. During any initial assessment or work with the client, it is important to make them the most important person in the room and focus on them. Skills and strategies to demonstrate this include:

- facing the person;
- maintaining eye contact (without staring);
- removing barriers such as desks/other equipment (during consultations);
- being interested and attentive to what the person is saying;
- being sensitive to your feelings and how these may be expressed (own facial expressions and body language);
- minimising distractions (e.g. ensuring mobile phones are switched off);
- leaning forwards slightly but not too far that you appear aggressive;
- keeping an open body and upright posture;
- reflecting warmth by demonstrating the core conditions (see Chapter 4, page 105);
- smiling naturally and being present; and avoiding fidgeting (Source: Lawrence & Barnett, 2006).

2. DURING THE WORK

The exercise professional will need to be able to adapt their working style to suit different client needs and the service that is available within their work setting. Some clients need regular meetings (weekly sessions or more frequent) with lots of support and encouragement, and may be more dependent on specific support interventions. Others will be more inclined towards self-management and will only need occasional meetings to discuss their progress. Active listening and questioning can be used to explore the client's needs and to check that these are being met. It is essential that the exercise professional is reflective and creative so that they can adapt their way of working to accommodate different needs (Source: Lawrence & Barnett, 2006).

3. ENDING THE WORK

When the work is due to end, the exercise professional should review the client's progress with them (this may involve reassessment) and identify how they can move forward and support and manage their own activity plan. Once again, active listening and questioning can be used. The exercise professional can use these skills to explore how the client feels about their progress and the work ending. They can also highlight any additional support that is available if it is needed (re-referral or exit pathways – e.g. other exercise sessions available when the working contract has ended, if the programme is part of a referral scheme etc.) and/or identify coping strategies that the client has established to manage their change (internal and external, etc.). All records that relate to the work with the client should be stored securely and maintained for future reference (Source: Lawrence & Barnett, 2006).

COMMUNICATION SKILLS
QUESTIONING

Asking appropriate questions can be an effective method for gathering information from the client. However, there can sometimes be a tendency to ask too many questions, which may block some clients from speaking if they feel they are under interrogation. Asking too many questions may also prevent active listening to what the client is saying as the exercise professional may be focused more on asking the questions as opposed to really listening and hearing the client's responses.

There are different types of questions that exercise professionals can use to gather information from their clients.

Open questions are most effective for gathering information in greater depth. When asked in the presence of the core conditions, open questions will generally enable the client to relax and will encourage them to speak openly. Open questions are those that that begin with the words: What? Who? How? Where? Why? When? How? For example: 'How did you feel after the last session?' and 'What types of activity do you like doing?'

Further information can then be gathered by using **probing questions** to encourage the client to expand on their initial response, or by using **focusing questions** to inquire more closely about specific responses that may help to define the problem more clearly. For example:

- Probing: 'Could you explain that?' or 'Tell me more about what you like about walking?' or 'Have you ever experienced that sensation before?'
- Focusing: 'Tell me more about the pain in your joint,' or 'Where exactly are you feeling the discomfort?' or 'What does that sensation in your chest feel like?'

ACTIVE LISTENING

Listening and hearing what the client is saying is a real skill and requires practice and much empathy on behalf of the exercise professional. It also requires the presence of the other core conditions (see Chapter 4, page 105). Active listening can be demonstrated in the following ways:

- Making some acknowledgement as the client speaks, for example, nodding the head, making eye contact, or saying yes or another sound (ummm, uh huh, etc.) that emphasises that they are being heard.
- Summarising what the client has said using your own language and using a questioning style so that they are able to correct anything misheard, for example, 'Am I hearing you say that you feel anxious before you arrive at the session?'
- Reflecting back what the client says by reading between the lines, for example, Client: '...and the doctors are just so insensitive.' Helper: 'Seeing other clients with cancer as you travelled with them today made you feel scared?' Client: 'Yes'.
- Asking questions if you do not understand or if you need further information from the client, for example: 'Would you tell me more about that so I can get a better picture?'

BARRIERS TO LISTENING

Even when we think we listen attentively, we need to be aware of other blocks that can occur.

Relating everything to yourself

One common block is relating everything to yourself and your own experience. This takes the focus off the person and back to you, for example, 'Yes, I find it difficult to make time to relax as well.' This may be true, but it is not useful for helping the person explore their difficulties.

Thinking about the next question

Another block to listening can be thinking about the next question you want to ask your client while they are still answering your previous question. If you are spending time thinking about your next question, you are not listening to what they are saying in the here and now! You may also be switching off to some vital information they are giving you.

Daydreaming

A further block is switching off and letting your mind daydream as the person speaks. If this happens it is far more respectful to apologise, acknowledge this and ask the client to repeat what they were saying.

Internal judgments

Making internal judgements on what the client has said will block you from hearing what the client is saying. Internally judging your client as unmotivated, lazy, a complainer, a nuisance, etc. also blocks your ability to be able to offer help, support and resolve difficulties.

Interrupting

Interrupting and giving advice when the person is speaking is another block to listening that needs to be avoided. For example, if the client says they struggle to find time to exercise, telling them what they should do to make time is not hearing the struggle they present. It is more helpful to acknowledge the struggle they present and then ask if they would like to explore different ways to overcome their struggle. It may be that they do not want to, or that they are not ready to change.

Being unempathic

Ignoring any expression of emotion and responding with shallow, unempathic comments is also unhelpful. For example, 'Well, we all find that difficult,' or 'It could be worse'. These comments draw attention away from what the person is experiencing and are quite dismissive. Exploration of these emotions may be crucial for identifying ways for them to move forward and resolve the issues presented for positive change.

Other blocks to listening

Further blocks to listening may include personal factors such as:

- Tiredness and personal stress.
- Individual differences (culture, gender, age, etc.).
- Having experiences too similar to those the person is presenting and thus, relating everything back to yourself.
- Not being able to relate to the person's experience. For example, a person complaining about not having time to exercise because they have children. If you do not have children, it may be more difficult to empathise.

CHANNELS OF COMMUNICATION

Communication is the process by which we both send and receive information and by which we can influence or be influenced by another person. For communication to be successful, it needs to be 'two-way' with both parties engaged and actively taking part in the process. Petty (2004) suggests that the chain of communication involves the four stages shown in figure 6.2.

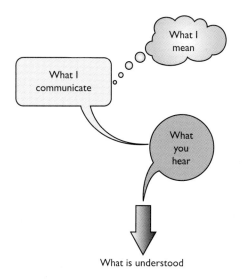

Figure 6.2 Stages of communication

Any 'break or block' within the communication chain may have significant effects on the message that is interpreted. The message sent and the message received may be affected by both conscious processes (those we are aware of) and also unconscious processes (those that are out of our current awareness).

Any discrepancy between what we say and how we feel will usually be communicated one way or another. The response we get from our communication may actually tell us more about what we are communicating than what we say, or how we choose to express it, at a conscious level. The more conscious we can be of our communication processes (including the body language we use) and the responses we receive from the recipient/s of our communication, the more potential we have to develop our communication skills.

Verbal communication
Language

To promote effective communication we need to use vocabulary that is appropriate to the person with whom we are communicating. The language people are comfortable using may be related to their educational background, their social class, country of origin and also the region within which they live.

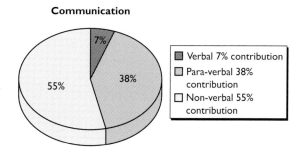

Figure 6.3 Contribution of different channels to overall communication

Table 6.1	Channels of communication		
Channel	**Verbal**	**Para-verbal**	**Non-verbal**
Examples	• What we say • Language we use • Words we speak or write • Jargon/terminology	• How we say things • Voice tone • Accent • Voice volume	• Body language • Posture and gestures • Eye contact and movements • Facial expressions • Proximity/closeness

Simple, non-technical language is usually more accessible to everyone and is therefore effective at communicating the message we want heard. The use of excessive terminology or intellectualising can be both confusing, intimidating, disorientating and can alienate some listeners, creating an instant block to the communication process. Colloquial or slang language should be avoided as it can be interpreted differently.

Jargon

All professions have aspects of jargon. In the exercise and fitness environment, technical muscle names are used (e.g. pectorals, instead of chest), muscle names are shortened (e.g. pecs) and choreography may be given specific names. If a person is unfamiliar with the jargon, the intended message will not be communicated, which can be both frustrating and disheartening. The use of simple and accessible language and/or explaining jargon will assist communication.

Para-verbal communication
Voice volume and tone

Voice volume and intonation can reflect our interest/emotion. Voice volume will need to be adapted to suit specific environments so that what we say is heard. A further consideration is that within different cultures/countries, volume and intonation can have a different meaning and affect. In the UK, shouting or speaking loudly can often be perceived as a sign of aggression and this can be distressing for some people. In other countries (India), quieter speech is accepted as a sign of politeness. In other countries (the USA) louder speech can be perceived as more natural practice. Awareness of body language and facial expressions used with specific intonations will also impact how communication is received.

Accent

In most countries and cultures there are a range of regional accents. Words spoken can be shortened and pronounced differently with the emphasis on different letters. The main consideration for persons with a strong regional accent or who knowingly shortens words would be to choose consciously to speak slightly slower and attend to pronunciation to assist communication.

Body language – the non-verbal channel

Most of our body language is spontaneous and outside of our conscious awareness. It often transmits the 'truth' (congruency) in relation to what we are feeling or thinking inside. Boyes (2005:9) suggests: '...what is not said verbally is often said non-verbally'. The most effective communicators are those who are most aware of and able to manage their body language to maximise the 'effect' of their message.

Body posture

Different body postures send different messages. An open posture, where we face the person and maintain an open and upright stance, will usually send a positive message. It usually demonstrates a willingness to be vulnerable and exposed/open to the other person. A closed posture, where our arms are folded and we stand facing slightly away from the person, may reflect that we perceive the other person as a threat or are uncomfortable with them in some way (Boyes, 2005:24).

Our posture can also reflect our interest in what is being said and also the attention we are paying to the person. If we face them, we are demonstrating they have our full attention. If we face them side on or face away from them, it reflects that we are distracted and no longer interested.

Facial expression

The face is perhaps the centre of all non-verbal communication (Boyes, 2005:31). The facial expressions we use as we speak can contain a whole array of messages, which may be unconscious to us but noticeable to others. We have over 90 muscles in the face, so it is unlikely that we will ever be able to control all of them. However, a wrinkle of the nose or a wink of an eye will send a message to the recipient.

Eyes and eye contact

The famous artist Leonardo da Vinci expressed that the eyes are the mirror to a person's soul (Boyes, 2005:32). The eyes reveal our true feelings. It is easier to spot if someone is feeling sad even if they say they are feeling okay. The eyes give away the real emotion and most of us can 'sense' the reality of the other person, whether we trust these intuitive feelings, or not. In addition, someone who is angry and expresses 'I'm fine' usually gives away their true feeling through their eyes.

One consideration, when working with persons with some mental health conditions may be the impact of their psychotropic medication and for some, the misuse of substances. Both of these can give the eyes a glazed appearance.

The amount of eye contact we give to another person may also reflect both how well we know them and how effectively we are relating to, or communicating with them. However, as with all body language, eye contact is bound by specific rules, which include intimacy levels with the other person, age, gender and culture.

Staring is considered threatening, aggressive and rude across cultures. Giving someone the 'eyeball' while telling them off is a way of expressing power, rank and control. From a gender perspective, women usually use more eye contact than men. Boyes (2005:34) suggests that women use eye contact to express involvement and interest, whereas men use it to indicate dominance and authority. Eye contact is sometimes viewed as a sexual invitation. Muslim women usually avoid direct eye contact with men.

The direction of gaze is also thought to reflect different intelligences – looking to the right is thought to indicate a lower visual and higher scientific imagination, whereas, looking to the left is thought to indicate a more artistic imagination (Boyes, 2005:35).

Eye movement has also been explored at a deeper level by neuro-linguistic programming (NLP) experts who suggest that specific eye movement patterns are true for most people.

- Moving the eyes to the left and down reflects own self-talk.
- Moving eyes to the right and down reflects connection with feelings/emotion.
- Moving the eyes upward and left or right indicates visual imaging.
- Moving the eyes sideways and right or left indicates auditory awareness – remembering what someone has said or thinking about what they will say.

Gestures

The movements of our hands, arms, legs, feet and head add to the communication. Consider raising the hand in front with the palm facing towards the person. Without using words, this passes the message for the person to stop! A thumbs up usually indicates that something is good and a simple crossing of the fingers means a wish for good luck. Stamping the foot or clenching the fists may indicate an expression of frustration, moving the hands and lowering the arms a lot may reflect expressiveness or anxiety depending on one's perspective.

A further thought for consideration is across cultures gestures can have different meanings. In the UK, the thumb and forefinger touching is used to give an 'OK' signal. In Brazil and the Middle East this gesture has a totally different and less polite meaning. In Italy and Greece, gesturing with hands during conversation reflects what is generally perceived as expression and passion. However, the quantity of gestures does not necessarily infer the emotion of the person. Some people gesticulate a lot as they speak to assist communication. Persons who are unable to communicate verbally (deaf or partial hearing) may use sign language (BSL or variations) to communicate.

When listening to another person, being aware and sensitive to the gestures they use can assist with communication and can reflect attention. In some instances, raising awareness to these gestures (if appropriate) can be useful to explore what is being said. For example, in a coaching situation, a person who is telling you they think they can do something but shaking their head (unconsciously) from right to left (expressing 'no') may be better prepared if they are able to become aware of and explore their head shaking. The mismatch between their words and gestures may mean that at some level they do not believe in their ability. However, in some cultures (Iran, Greece and Turkey) shaking the head can actually mean 'yes' (Boyes, 2005:28).

Proximity/personal space

The closeness at which we stand to people will also affect communication. Each person will have their own comfort zone for intimacy with others. Usually, the closer we stand to someone, the more intimate the relationship or the happier we are to develop intimacy with that person. For example, cuddling and comforting someone is an expression of personal intimacy.

Some factors that influence our personal space boundaries include physical stature, culture, topic of conversation, personality, gender, age, attraction and environment (e.g. in crowded places, our personal space boundaries are pushed but this is accepted, whereas, in a non-crowded environment, having someone stand very close to us may threaten our personal space and create feelings of discomfort).

A further consideration is that while one person may want to develop intimacy the other person may not. In professional environments, boundaries of role and ethical behaviour should be considered. Some vulnerable people can be less aware of boundaries and may behave more intimately and sometimes inappropriately for the situation. It is essential that the professional person can be respectful but also assertive with these boundaries, to protect themselves (e.g. from any potential allegations of abuse) and the vulnerable person, with whom they arc working by mirroring appropriate boundaries assertively.

COMMUNICATION STYLES

In reality we communicate using a variety of the styles described in table 6.2. The key is to be aware of which style we use predominately and in which situations and with which people. We can then choose to change the way we communicate, or not.

Table 6.2	Communication styles (adapted from Phelps & Austin, 1997)			
	Assertive	**Aggressive**	**Passive**	**Manipulative**
Position	I'm OK You're OK	You're not OK I'm OK	I'm not OK You're OK	You're not OK, but I will let you think you are OK
Personal power	Shares power and willing to be vulnerable	Controls and dominates to have power	• Helpless victim • Gives power to others • Uses guilt to control	Uses deceit to gain control and power
How others feel	• Respect • Inspired • Acceptance	• Fear • Humiliation • Hurt	• Guilty • Lose respect • Abused	• Suspicious • Confused • Manipulated
Courage	Willing to deal with difficulty and pain	Attacks and blames others	Does not stand up for self	Feigns other emotions to cover own fear
Outcome	Peace of mind	Lonely and bitter	Martyrdom – life is hard	Loss of trust and respect

Assertive communication

Being assertive requires expressing and acting on your own rights as a person while respecting the same rights in other people. Bayne et al., (1998) indicates that every person's assertive rights include:

- being treated with respect;
- expressing their thoughts, feelings, values and opinions;
- saying 'no' without feeling guilty;
- being successful;
- making mistakes;
- changing their mind;
- saying they don't understand;
- asking for what they want;
- deciding whether they are responsible for another person's problem or not; and
- choosing not to assert themselves.

These rights apply equally to all people, and all communication should aim to maintain both respect of self and respect of the other person as well. For example, expressing one's own opinion and values to discredit or hurt another person or without consideration to how these opinions impact the other person is not respectful or assertive. It can be seen as aggressive or manipulative communication, used to control, dominate or manipulate the other person. On the other hand, not expressing certain thoughts and our true feelings can be seen as passive communication, and may be a sign that we are giving our power away.

When working towards assertive communication, it is essential to be realistic. Some guidelines are:

- Do your best, it may not always be perfect. Other people may not always respond asser-tively back, nor will they always appreciate your assertions.
- Sometimes being assertive will not achieve the desired outcome – getting what we want.
- In some situations and with some people it may not be easy to be assertive and in some situations we may choose not to be assertive.
- The positive thing is, you can always try again (Phelps & Austin, 1997).

A strategy for assertive communication
- Decide what you want to achieve from the communication and what needs to be expressed, with respect to all persons involved.
- State clearly and specifically what you want to achieve and use 'I' statements ('I think' or 'I feel') to take ownership of thoughts and feelings.
- Support what you say with the corresponding body language, voice tone and vocabulary.

- Stay focused and stick to the agenda, without being sidetracked or manipulated. You can deal with other issues later.
- Listen to the other person – they have a right to their point of view.
- Aim for a win-win situation (cooperation).

SUMMARY POINTS
You should now be able to:

- Name the main stages of the working alliance.
- Describe the main communication at each stage of the alliance.
- Recognise different communication skills (active listening and questioning).
- Appreciate other factors that may influence the effectiveness of communication.
- Differentiate assertive communication from other styles of communication.

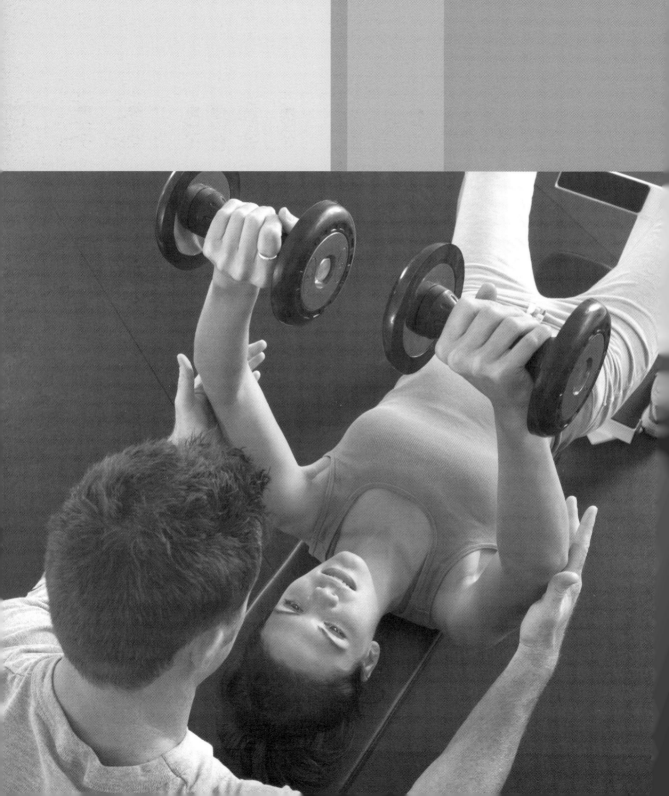

PART **THREE**

WORKING WITH CLIENTS

Exercise and physical activity are interventions that may help people to manage and improve their mental health. There are many other interventions that will be part of a holistic treatment plan and other qualified professionals will manage these.

The aim of this part is to clarify the role, responsibilities and boundaries for the exercise professional working with persons with mental health conditions. This section also provides information on making initial assessments to identify client needs and discusses considerations for planning and delivering physical activity and exercise sessions for this client group.

Case study

'Amber had reached a stage in her life where she was unable to leave the house to do anything – even putting the bins out. One of her friends spoke to me and asked if we could contact her to tell her about the scheme. After many phone calls, initially with her speaking about life in general, she eventually came to see us. The starting point consisted of me meeting her in the car park and walking and talking on the way to the gym office. Slowly and steadily and after many tears, we have built up to a 30–40 minute routine. Occasionally she relapses and I make sure to phone her and it does take some encouragement to talk her into coming back. Sometimes, if the gym is busy, we will go for a walk or go through a simple circuit of exercises in the studio. I am sure she will keep it up and that the results will keep showing.'

– Hannah Francis, Tenby Leisure Centre, Pembrokeshire County Council

ROLES, RESPONSIBILITIES AND BOUNDARIES

7

The primary role of the exercise professional is to ensure that their working practice (behaviour and actions) adheres to the code of ethical practice. A copy of the code of ethical practice is available from the register of exercise professionals (REPs) at www.exerciseregister.org.

When working with specialist groups (mental health, obesity, diabetes, etc.) the exercise professional may be required to work alongside other professionals, as part of a multi-disciplinary team. They are not expected to fulfil the roles and responsibilities of the other professionals who may be engaged in a client's treatment plan, which may include a GP, psychiatrist, counsellor, occupational therapist, physiotherapist, etc.

OBJECTIVES
By the end of this chapter you should be able to:

- define the role of the exercise professional;
- discuss the responsibilities and boundaries of the exercise professional role when working with clients;
- recognise the stages of the teaching cycle, which outlines areas of responsibility;
- recognise the role of reflective practice as a tool for continued professional development;
- discuss ethical practice and legal responsibilities, including reporting mechanisms and procedures; and
- recognise the signs and symptoms of risk (suicide, self-harm, psychotic episode and panic attacks) and identify sources for support and additional training for managing these areas.

Within all working roles, there are a number of responsibilities – these are usually listed and form part of a job description and may vary between different organisational settings. For example, an exercise professional working in a secure or hospital based setting may well have more additional responsibilities and boundaries than an exercise professional who is working as part of an exercise referral scheme or within a leisure club setting.

THE TEACHING CYCLE
The teaching cycle provides a framework that offers an overview of the main areas of responsibility for the exercise professional (see Figure 7.1).

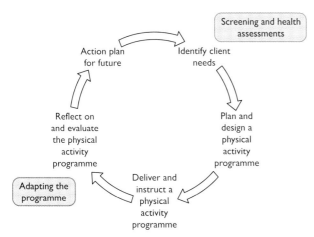

Figure 7.1 The teaching cycle

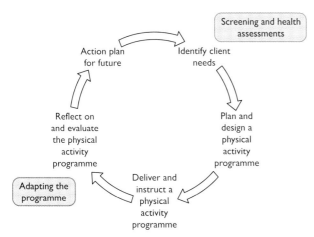

At each stage of the teaching cycle, there will be specific areas of responsibility and things for the exercise professional to consider and act upon.

IDENTIFY CLIENT NEEDS

Consideration should be given to:

- screening and informed consent (PAR-Q, interviews, providing information, such as referral or deferral, etc.);
- health assessments (heart rate, blood pressure and anthropometric measurements, such as hip, waist and BMI, etc.), body composition and functional ability;
- physical fitness assessments when appropriate (cardiovascular fitness, muscular fitness, flexibility, etc.);
- collecting personal information (client motivations, lifestyle, physical activity history, fitness goals, barriers to exercise, commitment, readiness to change, etc.);
- agreeing the working contract (number of sessions, cost, times, cancellations, etc.);

- establishing a working alliance and building rapport with the client; and
- maintaining communication with other health professionals involved in the client's treatment plan (exercise referral coordinators, physio-therapists, occupational therapists, community mental health teams, GPs, etc.).

PLANNING AND DESIGNING A PROGRAMME

Consideration should be given to the:

- setting (day care centre, community based, secure unit, hospital, leisure facility, etc.);
- environment (indoor, outdoor, gym, pool, space available, temperature, terrain, obstacles, etc.);
- type of equipment used, specific to the environment (water-based equipment, CV or RT machines, steps, bands, free weights, environmental equipment, portable equipment, etc.);
- type of clothing for both instructor and client that is appropriate to the environment (indoor and outdoor, including footwear) and appropriate for the activity;
- individual (programming to meet specific needs); and
- health and safety considerations specific to the individual, environment and equipments used (e.g. risk assessment and management, support of carers, unit staff).

DELIVER AND INSTRUCT A PROGRAMME

Consideration should be given to:

- interpersonal skills (communication style and skills, appearance, etc);

- teaching strategies (demonstration, explanation, questioning, monitoring intensity, observation, alternatives, gathering feedback, etc.);
- exercise and approaches (the training approaches to be used for all components of fitness using different exercise modalities, such as walking, cycling, etc.);
- session structure (duration, intensity and type of activity and exercise included for all components, such as the warm-up, main session, cool down); and
- progressions and regressions (adapting different activities and exercises to meet specific needs of individuals, environment, equipment, etc.)

REFLECTIVE PRACTICE AND EVALUATION

Consideration should be given to:

- gathering feedback from the client/s during and after the session;
- gathering feedback from other professionals involved in the client's care plan (psychiatrist, occupational therapist, etc.), e.g. effectiveness and appropriateness;
- gathering information from self (evaluating own practice, e.g. personal strengths and areas to develop);
- gathering information from other sources (a mentor or experienced exercise professional working with this population, etc.);
- reflective practice, which is an essential part of any professional's continued development. To become better at what we do, we need to reflect on and evaluate our practice. The exercise professional needs to be able to:
  - reflect on action (look back on the effectiveness of the session delivered; look back

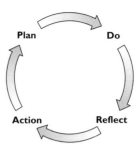

Figure 7.2 The reflective cycle (adapted from the work of Kolb (in Petty, 2004:147))

at the end of a full programme or course of sessions, and
- reflect in action (be aware of the effectiveness of interventions during their work and make adaptations as and when necessary – Boud et al., 1985).

Kolb (in Petty, 2004) provides a simple four-stage approach that provides a model for reflective practice (see Figure 7.2):

1 Planning – this is what I intended to do and why.
2 Delivery – this is what I did and what happened (descriptive statements).
3 Evaluation – this is what I think about what I did and what happened and my judgements about the experience (evaluative statements).
4 Action plan – this is what I will do next time.

ACTION PLANNING

Consideration should be given to:

- continued professional development to improve practice (skills, knowledge and attitudes);
- reading, further research and developing resources;

- working with a mentor and/or supervisor;
- attendance to additional training and workshops; and
- taking additional qualifications.

SUMMARY

In summary, the main responsibilities of the exercise professional are to:

- gather information to initially assess the client (screening);
- negotiate a working contract;
- establish a working alliance and build rapport with the client;
- maintain communication with other health professionals involved in the treatment plan (exercise referral coordinators, GPs, etc.);
- plan safe and effective exercise programmes;
- deliver safe and effective exercise programmes and adapt when appropriate;
- reflect on their practice and evaluate their planning and delivery; and
- maintain safe and ethical practice and work within the specific codes of practice (available on the REPs website).

The occupational descriptors for specific occupations within exercise and fitness (gym instructor, exercise to music instructor, personal trainer, exercise referral instructor, etc.) are available on the REPs website: www. exerciseresgister.org.

PROFESSIONAL BOUNDARIES

There are clear boundaries to every role in any profession. Boundaries ensure we work safely and

ethically and in the best interest of the client, the organisation and ourselves equally. It is not the role of the exercise professional to be a doctor, therapist, counsellor, friend or surrogate parent. However, there may be aspects of these other roles that are essential within the professional relationship and which may support the development of a working alliance between an exercise professional and client. There may be times when the exercise professional needs to:

- actively listen (act as counsellor);
- provide information (act as a teacher);
- offer different strategies and interventions (act as a creative and strategic planner);
- offer motivation and support (act as a nurturer and supporter);
- help the client to establish goals (act as a goal setter); and
- challenge the client, testing and checking their reality, perception, beliefs (act as a liberator, who helps the client to build independence) in relation to exercise myths and benefits.

The key is for the exercise professional to be aware and respectful of the boundaries of their role, such as:

- being friendly and approachable without crossing the boundary into being a friend;
- being willing to listen without crossing the boundary into being a counsellor or therapist;
- having an awareness of signs and symptoms of a condition without crossing the boundary into medical expert and diagnosing and/or prescribing; and
- providing information without crossing the boundary of being the expert in all areas;

- offering creative strategies without moving into a parental role and being required to solve all of the client's problems.

CONFIDENTIALITY
PERSONAL CONFIDENTIALITY

When working with clients' it is essential to maintain personal confidentiality. It is recommended that specific details, such as home or work addresses or telephone numbers, are not disclosed. It is also not advisable to disclose information about one's personal life circumstances or family or friends, as this is potentially crossing the boundary into becoming a friend.

On occasion, a client may want to get closer to you and enquire about you, especially if you are helping them. However, becoming too friendly may cause problems or an unnecessary attachment. It may also cause resentment among other clients if working in a group situation, where other group members may perceive one person as being favoured.

Maintaining this boundary can sometimes feel hard. However, once a boundary is removed, it will be difficult to reinstate it without some resentment being experienced, which can block rapport and the relationship. The aim is not to be unnecessarily secretive or create a barrier for communication but to maintain your own personal boundaries that need to be in place to protect yourself.

Ultimately, it is up to the individual exercise professional to decide how much information they choose to disclose to clients. The exercise professional code of ethical practice and the ethical practice guidelines of other professions (e.g. *BACP Code of Ethics and Practice for Counsellors* and the codes of practice for other health professions) will offer further guidance on this matter.

CLIENT CONFIDENTIALITY

When working with persons with mental health issues, it is essential to ensure strict confidentiality. Any records that need to be maintained will be covered by specific laws, such as the Freedom of Information Act and Data Protection Act. All records that need to be maintained should be kept locked away with restricted access to specifically named personnel only. They will also need to be available for the person to review on request.

As an exercise professional, you should never engage in general conversation about the client with any other person or group. The only exception to this rule is that you may need to discuss specific issues with other professionals who are working with the client or supervising your own work. In these instances, the client's name may still need to remain confidential.

WORKING WITH OTHER PROFESSIONAL AGENCIES

In any workplace where you will be working with vulnerable people you will be asked to complete a disclosure form provided by the Criminal Records Bureau (CRB). CRB is an executive agency of the Home Office, which helps employers and volunteering organisations to make informed recruitment decisions and protect the vulnerable members of society. The CRB record is a confidential document that details an individual's criminal record, and where appropriate, if the person is banned from working with vulnerable adults or children.

WORKING CONTRACTS

The working contract is the arrangement for working together made between the client and the exercise professional. Some organisations will specify the duration and times for the contract. This is dependent on the set up of any specialist schemes that operate in the organisation and whether they have the support of funding and also expertise from other local organisations, for example, exercise on referral schemes, community mental health teams, other mental health groups, etc.

Short-term contracts

In many services a short-term contract (up to three months) is all that is available. Such short-term contracts can put you at a disadvantage, as they may demand that a more directive method of work is taken, meaning it will be difficult to develop a deeper working alliance with your client. You will also need to ensure that there are clear exit pathways that extend to the person beyond this initial contract. Without these pathways, exercise adherence may cease (Lawrence & Barnett, 2006).

Longer term contracts

In some services, longer term working contracts may be available (beyond three months). An advantage of longer term contracts is that the exercise professional can potentially develop a deeper working alliance with the client and can work in a more creative way, exploring and experimenting with different activities and types of programme.

A longer term contract can also provide more support to the person, especially if they struggle to implement the changes they desire. Longer term working may help the client to access and sustain the level of support and motivation they need to maintain the changes more permanently and independently. In reality, a lifetime of choosing unhealthy thinking patterns and unhealthy behaviours, attitudes and habits is unlikely to change overnight (Lawrence & Barnett. 2006).

One possible disadvantage of a longer term contract may be that the client becomes dependent on the helper or service. Within settings where exercise programmes are funded, some independence needs to be encouraged to promote sustainability of the project.

RISK ASSESSMENT

Risk assessment is a key responsibility for the exercise professional and other professionals who are working with the person. Initial screening and information gathering is an essential aspect of all working roles. It is the exercise professional's responsibility to provide safe and effective exercise or activity. Some contraindications for and reasons to delay exercise are explored in chapter 8 (see page 153).

Risk assessments may also uncover something that you believe may present a potential risk or danger to the person or others. Anything that causes you to feel uneasy or raises concern should be reported immediately to another health professional (in particular a member of unit staff or CMHT) who is familiar with the client and will be far better qualified to respond and act upon such information. It may evolve to be nothing, but it is better to be safe than sorry.

MEDICAL EMERGENCIES
PANIC ATTACKS

If an individual experiences a panic attack it can be very frightening for them and for anyone around them, including you. Panic attacks can share symptoms of other medical conditions such as a heart attack or asthma attack. The person may feel fine one minute and the next they are trembling, sweating, hyperventilating and experiencing palpitations. They may feel dizzy, fear they are dying, feel numbness or tingling and/or even experience chest pain. Some people who experience panic attacks will carry a crisis card and others do not, so if there is any doubt about the person's symptoms, you should call the emergency services. The following tips from Mental Health First Aid (MHFA) offer good advice for coping with a panic attack (www.mhfa.com.au/firstaid. shtml):

- Stay calm!
- Reassure them constantly and tell them the panic attack will pass and they will be OK.
- If possible, move them to a quiet place where there are no bystanders.
- Encourage them to breathe slowly and calmly – it can be useful to exaggerate your own breathing and mirror deeper, slower breathes. Likewise speaking slowly and staying relaxed will help them to return to a calmer state.
- Let them speak and listen to any fears with empathy.
- Continue to reassure them.
- Stay with them until help arrives.

Remaining calm and non-judgemental is key to successful defusing of difficult situations. At no time should you display impatience, anger or pity as this may exacerbate the situation. Similarly your choice of words is crucial: telling someone to 'pull yourself together', 'calm down' or 'don't be silly' often has the opposite effect.

PSYCHOTIC EPISODE/MENTAL HEALTH CRISIS

It is rare, but not impossible, for someone with depression or anxiety to experience a more serious or psychotic episode. A mental health crisis may occur when a person feels suicidal, or may be having an anxiety attack or an acute stress reaction.

If this happens, the individual may have lost touch with reality and can be extremely distressed and, on occasion, violent. The following course of action is recommended:

- If someone is at risk of being hurt, call the emergency services.
- Do not approach the person if it is unsafe to do so.
- If you judge it safe, approach the person and introduce yourself, explaining why you are present and offering to help.
- Remain courteous and non-threatening, but be honest and direct.
- Listen to the person in a non-judgemental way.
- Avoid confrontation at all costs – do not confront them or argue with them, even if they are saying irrational things, be prepared to 'agree to differ' with the person's perspective and accept their 'reality'.
- Clarify and address what the person sees as the major issues first (not what you, the helper, see as the major concerns).
- Do not attempt to manhandle the person or force him/her to do anything in particular.

- Encourage/assist the person to receive professional mental health help.
- Finally, if the incident was traumatic for you, or you feel anxious or distressed, discuss these issues with a friend or a professional service.

SUICIDE

Suicide is a risk for many persons suffering with mental health conditions. The NHS (2010) and Rethink (2010) indicate research that has found:

- 30 per cent of people with schizophrenia will attempt suicide at least once;
- 1 in 10 people with schizophrenia will commit suicide;
- between 30–40 per cent of people with schizoaffective disorder will attempt suicide during their lifetime; and
- 10 per cent of people with schizoaffective disorder will succeed.

The warning signs

What follows is a list of warning signs that can indicate that people with depression and schizophrenia are considering suicide. The person:

- is making final arrangements (giving away possessions, making a will or saying goodbye to friends);
- is talking about death or suicide (direct statements such as, 'I wish I was dead,' or indirectly, 'Wouldn't it be nice to go to sleep and never wake up,');
- is self-harming (cutting arms or legs or burning themselves with cigarettes); and/or
- has a sudden lifting of mood (this could mean that a person has decided to commit suicide and feels better because of their decision).

The NHS (2010) recommends that if you notice any of the warning signs you should:

- ensure your own safety;
- get professional help for the person, such as a crisis resolution team (CRT) or the duty psychiatrist at your local A&E department;
- let the person know that they are not alone and that you care about them;
- offer support in finding other solutions to their problems;
- stay with them, if the danger is immediate; and
- remove all means of suicide (e.g. medication, sharp objects).

It may be necessary for the exercise professional to undertake additional training for the management of risk (suicide, self-harm etc.). Applied Suicide Intervention Skills Training (ASIST) is a two-day training course to teach people how to intervene if a person is suicidal. The course is delivered in Wales in conjunction with Mind Cymru (see www.livingworks.net).

SELF-HARM

Self-harm is a frequently encountered response to emotional or mental distress. It can take many forms and perhaps the more familiar is that of a person cutting or injuring themselves on purpose. However, taking an overdose, misusing drugs and alcohol, smoking, overeating, developing an eating disorder or staying in an abusive relationship are all forms of self-harm and may be overlooked or ignored if a perceived 'greater' mental health condition is present. The majority of individuals who self-harm are young women, however, men are increasingly at risk of self-harming behaviour, particularly as an outlet for otherwise suppressed emotions.

In response to pain (self-inflicted or other), the body releases endorphins, which can give a lift to mood. One explanation for self-harming is that the endorphins offer an alternative short-term fix for managing uncomfortable feelings. Another reason for self-harming may include a belief of 'being in control'. Certainly, when a person resorts to self-harming they have lost any love or respect for their own self and being and should therefore be encouraged to seek help through counselling and therapy.

The majority of people who self-harm have undergone difficult, painful or abusive experiences as a child or adolescent. Self-harm can be a coping strategy, a form of release or a distraction at times when emotions are overwhelming. For some it may be an attempt to communicate feelings to others (a cry for help) or a way of having some control in life. It may also be a form of self-punishment or the expression of self-hatred.

Most people will attempt to hide the results of self-harm by wearing oversized or clothes that cover their body, which may seem inappropriate in the exercise environment. The person will not take these clothes off, even if they get very hot or sweaty during exercise, and as the exercise professional you need to ensure intensity is at a level that accounts for this.

It may be that as people get to know and trust you they no longer cover up the evidence of self-harm and this can be very distressing when you see it for the first time. A key consideration is not to react with shock (not always easy!) and/or to stare.

RECORD KEEPING

Another essential responsibility that is governed by both legal and professional requirements is to maintain appropriate records. Specific requirements may vary in different work environments, so it is advisable to check what these are for settings and workplaces. Client records that need to be maintained will usually include:

- a referral letter from their GP or other health professional;
- screening and health information (PAR-Q, etc.);
- session records (registers, programme cards, lesson plans, evaluations, etc.);
- progress reports that need to be provided for medical and other health professionals to review; and
- incident and accident report forms (when applicable).

STANDARDS OF RECORDS

Any record needs to be easily reviewed by other related health professionals (as appropriate). They should therefore:

- be clear and legible (typed or neat handwriting);
- be informative and succinct to provide feedback to other professionals;
- list the date and time of any information that is updated;
- have the name and signature of the person making the entry (with counter signatories for trainee staff);
- provide professional and descriptive information, and not evaluative (value-based, e.g. good, poor, etc.) or judgmental information about the person's way of being or behaviour.

For example, 'X was fidgeting in their chair during the warm-up' (which is descriptive and factual), as opposed to, 'X was being awkward' (which is evaluative and judgmental); and

- corrections and updates should be clear and signed by the person making the amendment.

SUMMARY POINTS

You should now be able to:

- Explain some of the responsibilities and boundaries of the exercise professional when working with clients.
- Name the stages of the teaching cycle.
- Explain different responsibilities of the exercise professional at different stages of the teaching cycle.
- Describe ethical practice and the legal responsibilities of the exercise professional.
- Describe how the reflective practice model can be used.
- Recognise signs and symptoms for risk of suicide, self-harm, psychotic episode and panic attacks.
- Identify referral sources relating to these risk situations.
- Identify sources of additional training for managing these situations.

ASSESSING CLIENT NEEDS

8

This chapter reviews the information that needs to be gathered prior to planning a session and working with clients. It explores methods of gathering information and exclusion criteria.

OBJECTIVES

By the end of this section you should be able to:

- recognise the purpose of initial assessment as a way of gathering information to identify needs;
- recognise the information that needs to be gathered, with regard to physical, medical, psychological, lifestyle needs;
- recognise methods of gathering information;
- recognise the American College of Sports Medicine (ACSM) risk stratification criteria;
- recognise reasons for referral and deferral; and
- recognise a range of health and physical assessments.

REASONS FOR ASSESSMENT AND APPROPRIATENESS OF TESTS

If an exercise assessment is to be included, it is essential to be clear on the purpose of the assessment (reasons for including it) and ensure that the

assessment is appropriate and individualised (adapted, when necessary) to meet the needs of the client. All assessments should provide meaningful and useful information and offer a positive experience for the client.

Each assessment should be conducted by a person who is qualified and competent to carry out the assessments. When conducting assessments, the aim should be to involve the client as much as possible and provide a clear explanation about what assessments are being conducted and their purpose, and providing the client with the opportunity to ask questions.

INITIAL ASSESSMENT AND IDENTIFYING NEEDS

The main purpose of initial assessment is to gather information from the client and other agencies (GP, community mental health team, carer, psychiatrist or other referring service, etc.) to check the current health status of the client. The exercise professional will be responsible for:

- maintaining contact with the client and any referral agencies to gather information to assess the client's needs;

- identifying any barriers that may prevent participation;
- conducting a risk assessment; and
- negotiating a provisional contract of working.

The information that needs to be gathered includes the client's personal details, such as their name, address, emergency contac detailst, and also the contact details and signature of any referring agency (e.g. carer, GP, physiotherapist, social worker). More specific information may include that shown in figure 8.1.

REFERRAL AND DEFERRAL

The information shown in figure 8.1 can be used to identify any needs that will inform both the advice given and the exercise prescription provided by the exercise professional. It will determine whether the person:

- is **ready** to become more active, e.g. apparently healthy, with no identified risks;
- will need to be **referred** to a specialist professional, e.g. a GP, to gather additional medical information for clearance or a specialist

---

Physical

- Age
- Resting heart rate
- Blood pressure
- Height and weight, BMI
- Any additional support needs (carer, language support/communicator, BSL signer, etc.)

Medical

- Any current or previous medical conditions or physical health problems that may affect participation
- Medication taken (what taken, how long taken for and any recent changes)

Lifestyle

- Current and previous activity and exercise experience
- Previous exercise and activity problems (including likes and dislikes)
- Other behaviours (smoking, alcohol or use of other substances)

Psychological

- Self-efficacy and belief
- Motivation and readiness to make changes
- Expectations and goals
- Barriers/fears or concerns

Other

- Social and psychiatric history
- Whether the client has been sectioned (where appropriate) and which section. Whether this was voluntary, or not
- Whether the client is an in-patient or an out-patient?
- Any risk or precautions (behavioural problems, violence, self harm, suicide, etc.)
- Recommended activity

Figure 8.1 Information that can be gathered by an initial assessment

exercise instructor, for programme design and delivery (cardiac rehabilitation, etc.); or

- will need to **delay** participation, e.g. if unwell or presenting with a medical condition that meets exclusion criteria and requires medical clearance.

If any of the information listed in figure 8.1 is not available, it may be advisable to defer and delay participation, especially if there is any doubt (from self or client) regarding the safety of self, client or others. Figure 8.2 indicates the stratification of some physical and medical risks.

Clients with a moderate risk rating may be able to exercise at a low to moderate level of intensity (equivalent RPE 3–4 on the CR10 scale, see Chapter 9, page 169) without undergoing any further physical assessments. Exercising at a low to moderate intensity offers significantly lower risk than exercising at a high intensity. Low to moderate activity also promotes **adherence**, which is a primary goal for persons with mental health conditions.

Clients with a higher risk rating should be referred for clinical assessment and clearance prior to becoming more active.

INFORMATION GATHERING TOOLS

There are numerous ways of gathering information, which include:

- self-administered questionnaires (e.g. PAR-Q);
- written questionnaires completed with a medical professional (e.g. PARmedX, Warwick Edinburgh Mental Well-being Scale);
- Hospital Anxiety and Depression Scale;
- interview or verbal questions;
- observation;
- health assessments; and

- functional and physical assessments.

PAR-Q

The PAR-Q may be a less effective tool for gathering information from some persons with mental health conditions. The structure, layout and wording of the self-screening form may appear too formal and confusing. As an alternative, information can be gathered by the exercise professional verbally, using open questions (see page 130) and simplifying the language, or it can be gathered in advance from another health professional.

The questions asked on the PAR-Q often place too much emphasis on negative symptoms. For some people with mental health conditions, this can heighten their anxiety and may discourage participation for fear of exacerbating their existing conditions. Once again, verbal questioning (using open questions) can be used to enable the questionnaire to be phrased more positively.

In addition, some of the questions identified on the PAR-Q reflect symptoms that are experienced as a side effect from taking psychotropic medication (e.g. dizziness, high blood pressure, etc). Ideally, any information on medication being taken needs to be gathered in advance. Clients who respond 'Yes' to the questions should complete the PARmedQ continuation before participating.

Informed consent

Prior to any activity or pre-exercise assessment the person needs to provide their informed consent (National Quality Assurance Framework, 2001). This offers the exercise professional an opportunity to discuss the proposed pre-exercise assessment and/or planned physical activity programme. An informed consent document should be written and provide the following:

- Sufficient information, in accessible language
- An explanation of the purpose of the exercise assessment and/or programme
- A description of the components of the exercise assessment and/or programme
- An explanation of the possible risks, discomforts and benefits
- Clarification of the responsibilities of the client
- A reference to confidentiality and privacy
- An emphasis on the client's voluntary participation and right to change their mind
- The opportunity for the client to ask questions (questions and answers can be recorded)

Informed consent is not a legal waiver and if someone has not given sufficient information the document is not valid, even if it has been signed (NQAF, 2001).

Health measurements

These assessments form part of the first steps for checking whether the person should take part in physical activity and exercise.

Excessively high resting heart rate and excessively high blood pressure are a contra-indication for exercise. If these present, the person should delay activity until the symptoms are managed. Alternatively, a clinically supervised exercise programme may be required.

Resting heart rate

Resting heart rate is usually taken immediately after a long rest (e.g. sleep). It can enable detection of:

- normal heart rate 60–100bpm;
- bradycardia (slow heart rate) <60bpm;
- tachycardia (fast heart rate) >100bpm; and
- an irregular heart rate.

Exercise should be deferred or delayed if any of the following present:

- A resting heart rate of >100bpm. This is a contraindication for exercise and a client presenting this should be referred back to their GP.
- A client presenting with a slow resting heart rate. This should be assessed further. The client may be taking medication such as beta-blockers, which affects heart rate and in which case, the intensity of any activity will need to be reduced.
- A client presenting with a resting heart rate <40bpm or who is experiencing symptoms such as dizziness. The client should be advised not to exercise and referred back to their GP.

Heart rate is also affected by a number of other factors these include:

- Medications
- Stress or anxiety
- Eating
- Smoking
- Caffeine
- Temperature

Resting blood pressure

Resting heart rate is also taken after a period of rest. This assessment provides the opportunity to identify:

> **Low risk: Ready to become active without medical clearance**

- Men <45 years of age and women <55 years of age who are asymptomatic and meet **no more than one other risk factor:**
  - Family history of heart disease
  - Smoking
  - Hypertension
  - High cholesterol
  - Impaired fasting glucose
  - Obesity
  - Sedentary lifestyle

> **Moderate risk: Can participate in low to moderate intensity activity without medical clearance**

- Men ≥45 years of age and women ≥55 years or those who meet the threshold for **two or more risk factors:**
  - Family history of heart disease
  - Smoking
  - Hypertension
  - High cholesterol
  - Impaired fasting glucose
  - Obesity
  - Sedentary lifestyle

> **High risk: Requires medical clearance before starting a physical activity programme**

- **Individuals with one or more of the following signs and symptoms:**
  - Angina pain or discomfort
  - Shortness of breath at rest or with mild exertion
  - Dizziness or syncope
  - Othopnea (breathlessness (dyspnoea) occurring at rest in the recumbent position that is relieved by sitting upright) or paroxysmal nocturnal dyspnoea (breathlessness which usually begins 2–5 hours after going to sleep)
  - Ankle oedema
  - Palpitations or tachycardia
  - Intermittent claudication
  - Known heart murmur or know cardiovascular, pulmonary or metabolic disease (angioplasty, angina)
  - Cardiac (myocardial infarction, coronary artery bypass surgery, coronary angioplasty, angina)
  - Cerebrovascular (stroke, transient ischaemic attack)
  - Peripheral vascular disease
  - Pulmonary disease (chronic obstructive pulmonary disease/cystic fibrosis, asthma)
  - Metabolic disease (diabetes Type I and Type II), thyroid, renal or liver disease

Figure 8.2 ACSM risk stratification (ACSM, 2010:23)

- hypotension (when blood pressure is lower than normal). Hypotension is usually asymptomatic, however, some people may feel dizzy or faint when they stand up. This is referred to as postural hypotension and may be caused by a number of conditions or the effects of medication such as beta-blockers or diuretics;
- normal blood pressure (<120 systolic and <80 diastolic);
- pre-hypertension (120–139 systolic or 80–89 diastolic);
- stage 1 hypertension (140–159 or 90–99 diastolic); and
- stage 2 hypertension (>160 systolic or >100 diastolic). A systolic blood pressure of >180mmHg and a diastolic blood pressure of >100 mmHg is a **contraindication** for exercise and further physical assessments.

If the reading is higher than expected the measurement should be repeated at the end of the assessment (but before any other physical assessments that require exertion).

Psychological measurements

For persons with mental health conditions, subjective measures that relate to their perceived well-being and levels of motivation are arguably the most important. The ASCM (2010:176) presents a self-motivation assessment scale that can be used to determine the person's initial motivation and their proneness for non-compliance.

There are also other psychological assessment scales that can identify the person's starting mood, thoughts and feelings. These include the Warwick Edinburgh Mental Well-being Scale and the Hospital Anxiety and Depression Scale (HADS). These scales ask questions that relate to a person's levels of enjoyment, anxiety levels, mood, and functioning. When administered over time, they offer a way of measuring the individual's subjective experiencing, which may be influenced by them becoming more active. These assessment tools are only available from organisations that hold a license to use them and have gained permission from the copyright holders.

Physical assessments

Health-related physical assessments can be used to obtain further information from the client. Pre-exercise assessments (ACSM, 2005; Buckley & Jones, 2005) can be useful to:

- educate the client about their current levels of fitness;
- collect baseline information, which can be used to develop an exercise programme and tailor advice for daily activities;
- monitor progress and help motivate clients;
- assist risk stratification;
- gather useful information about a client's response to sub-maximal exercise including heart rate, rating of perceived exertion (RPE), etc.; and
- explore difficulties the client has in terms of carrying out the assessment including following instructions, motor skills and the influence of comorbidities.

Anthropometric measurements

These assessments include taking various measurements from which body composition can be estimated. They include height, weight and body mass index (BMI), waist circumference and skinfold measurements.

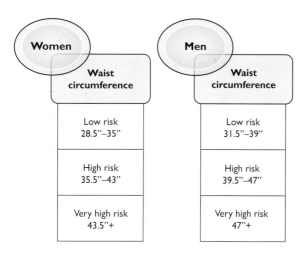

Figure 8.3 Waist circumference and risk (adapted from Bray, 2004, in ACSM, 2010:66)

The simplest of these assessments is to measure waist circumference. Body composition and, in particular, high body fat around the trunk or waist is recognised as increasing the risk of coronary heart disease and other health problems including high blood pressure, high cholesterol, diabetes (type II) and stroke (ACSM, 2010:62).

Waist circumference

Waist circumference is a slightly invasive assessment as it requires a physical measurement of the waist to be taken, which for some persons with low self-esteem may reinforce in them a feeling of 'not being OK'. Sensitivity to these issues should be considered prior to considering this assessment and guesstimate measures can be provided via observation as an alternative, albeit inaccurate, measurement. Figure 8.3 indicates measurements that offer higher risk.

Postural assessment

Optimal posture minimises the stress placed on the body tissues. Over a period of time poor posture may contribute to health problems such as tension headaches, joint problems, back pain and less effective breathing patterns.

Posture can be assessed using a number of observational tools such as a standard reference line and/or a simple checklist to check the position of body parts such as shoulder blade alignment, level of skin creases and asymmetry in muscle bulk (Norris, 2003). Identifying postural defects (lordosis, kyphosis, flat back, etc.) can enable the exercise professional to consider these within their planning. Any muscle imbalance contributing to poor posture can be addressed through reeducation and strengthening of postural muscles in conjunction with stretching exercises.

Other physical assessments

There are many other physical assessments that can be used to assess and monitor improvements in physical fitness (cardio-respiratory fitness, muscular strength, muscular endurance, flexibility, etc.). The appropriateness (including validity and reliability) of these assessments is discussed in the ACSM (2010) *Guidelines for Exercise Testing and Prescription*.

ONGOING ASSESSMENT AND REVIEW

The assessment process needs to be ongoing. Before every session it is important to reassess the client's readiness to exercise and monitor any changes in their health status. This may include:

- any other changes in their medical and mental health from initial assessment or the previous session;
- the person's response to previous exercise session such as excessive tiredness or discomfort;
- any incidence of chest pain or other physical symptoms, which may require referral or deferral; and/or
- the results/outcomes of any appointments and tests (with a GP or other health professionals).

It can be helpful to plan regular review dates to assess progress, discuss any concerns that the client has and identify ongoing support needs. Ongoing assessment enables the exercise professional to respond to the needs of the client, modify/adapt, regress or progress the programme as appropriate and support exercise adherence.

The process of information gathering, which includes pre-exercise screening and assessment, will enable the development of a more structured exercise programme or exercise prescription. It can also help to develop a strong foundation for encouraging long-term physical activity and behaviourial change.

For persons with mental health conditions, the most useful reference may well be the psychological measures and their perceived well-being. While less objective, these measures arguably have the most impact on the person and their adherence or reasons for non-compliance. Any improvements in physical fitness and health can be seen to some extent as an additional and bonus achievement.

SUMMARY POINTS

You should now be able to:

- State the purpose of gathering information.
- Give an example of when you may need to refer a client to another professional or advise them to defer exercise and activity to a later date.
- State the purpose of informed consent.
- Give an example of a questionnaire you may use when assessing a client initially.
- Identify some criterias for exclusion from exercise.
- State the purpose for using some basic health and physical assessments.

DESIGN, DELIVERY AND ADAPTATION

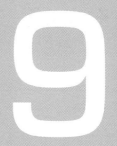

This chapter reviews the considerations for designing safe and effective activity and exercise intervention. It looks at a range of different working environments and types of activity and exercise intervention. It also revises basic delivery and teaching skills, methods for monitoring intensity and ways to progress and regress activities and exercises.

OBJECTIVES

By the end of this chapter you should be able to:

* recognise planning considerations and goal setting;
* describe different work environments and settings;
* recognise session structure;
* review a range of session types;
* discuss the merits of each session type for working with specific conditions with consideration to comorbidities/medications;
* review methods for monitoring intensity; and
* recognise methods for progressing and regressing different activities.

PRE-PLANNING CONSIDERATIONS

Prior to delivering any activity or exercise session, it is necessary to make the considerations shown in table 9.1.

All of these questions should be considered with regard to information gathered from individuals who will be attending. The purpose of the session should also be considered and specific goals and session outcomes established. These can be used as measures to check the effectiveness of the session and identify where adaptations need to be made.

WORKING ENVIRONMENTS

Exercise and physical activity can take place in a number of different environments, beyond the gym and studio. Providing exercise in different environments can promote accessibility and some environments have additional positive effects of mental health and well-being.

The outdoors and green exercise

Numerous exercise and activity programmes can be delivered in an outdoor environment. These include walking, gardening, climbing, tai chi, running, cycling, kite flying, circuit training, bootcamps, horse riding, rambling and conservation

Table 9.1		Planning considerations	Example considerations
Question		**Specific questions**	**Example considerations**
Who?	1a	How many will be attending?	Need to know for space and equipment
	1b	What are the specific needs of individuals?	Physical, medical and mental health needs all need to be considered
	1c	Have you taught them before?	Will help to assess with level – see 2b
	1d	Will you be teaching them again?	Need to consider progression
	1e	Have they exercised before?	Link to 2b
	1f	What support staff are available?	Consider number in group
What?	2a	What type of session?	Gym, exercise to music (ETM), chair, aqua, circuits. Is it a group session or one to one?
	2b	What will be the level of the class?	Fitness, skill, intensity
	2c	What resources do you need?	Stereo, mats, weights, chairs, etc.
Where?	3a	Where is the venue and is it a community, secure or sports facility setting?	Consider access, safety and 'friendliness'
	3b	Is there enough space for all?	May affect type of class
	3c	What resources are available?	Link to 2c and 5c
	3d	Have you worked there before, do you know where all the amenities are and what health and safety issues may you need to consider (fire exits, drill, etc.)?	If it is in a unit, you need to know their rules and systems. If working in a centre, ensure familiarity with the SOP and EAP. If in the community what else do you need to know?
	3e	Are there any access problems?	Do you need wheelchair access? Are the toilets accessible?
	3f	Will carers or helpers be available?	May be necessary to have others to help with unexpected situations
	3g	Where is the emergency contact and duty first aider?	Need full contact details and an additional first aider is advisable
When?	4a	Time of day/day of week	Consider timing of medications, other people who may be around
	4b	Length of session	Sessions may need to be much shorter to accommodate fitness and attention levels
How?	5a	How will you arrange the room?	Is there space for the session you want to run?
	5b	What teaching methods will you use?	How will you observe and what correction is appropriate?
	5c	What resources will you use? Do you need to create or buy resources (balls and bands, etc.)?	Do you have everything you need with you? Consider health and safety when using equipment
	5d	What ground rules will you need to establish/maintain?	Need to ensure that these are not off-putting but are acceptable to the group
	5e	What are your goals and aims? What are their goals and targets?	The session must reflect the aims and abilities of the group, not you
	5f	How will you monitor and record progress?	What type of notes are appropriate? Who will have access to these?

projects among others. There is also increasing evidence to suggest that exercising outdoors can have many positive benefits for mental health. Bird (2007) suggests that we have a connection to the natural outdoor environment and that we are more content and function more effectively when in this environment. This is known as the Biophilia theory.

Being in a natural environment can help the brain to recharge and refocus. The natural environment provides an escape and distraction for the brain from the daily routine and the tasks we concentrate on directly, which may be uninteresting and consequently require more brain energy. Being outdoors provides fascination and a more interesting focus for the brain. It requires little concentration and allows the brain to relax. This is known as Attention Restoration Theory, or ART (Bird, 2007).

There is also evidence to suggest that the body has an immediate positive physiological response to natural views, which include reduced blood pressure, reduced muscle tension and reduce heart rate (Psycho-physiological stress recovery theory. Bird 2007). Dr William Bird and the volunteering charity the British Trust for Conservation Volunteers (BTCV) set up 'Green Gyms' with the specific intention of attracting people to use the green, outdoor spaces to improve physical, emotional and mental well-being. Green Gyms are open to everyone and members meet at least once a week for between one and four hours' practical conservation or gardening work (an alternative to gym-based training). The benefits of green gyms and green exercise are shown below.

- It is a cost-effective method of improving physical and mental well-being.

- Outdoor programmes can provide exit routes for exercise referral schemes and other public health improvement strategies, e.g. mental health, obesity, etc.
- It can support corporate health by offering access to activity and exercise close to the workplace.
- It can offer opportunities for learning, e.g. conservation, which may increase potential employability.
- It promotes socialisation.
- It improves neighbourhoods and community areas.
- It can promote independence.

For more information, visit www.btcv.org.uk/display/greengym.

'Marvellous. Absolutely brilliant! Recommend it to anyone. If anyone else is suffering from depression, or stuck indoors, just give them a call. Just go for it, don't be afraid, just go for it. Cause I was scared, but I'm still here...'

– Client from Sustrans.
Bike it, Walk it project evaluation, 2009

Water-based exercise

For centuries, water has provided a medium for the sport and recreation of different civilisations. It is well documented that the ancient Greeks and Romans used water for a variety of purposes. These included assisting with the alleviation of fatigue and low spirits, promoting cleanliness and enhancing a general feeling of well-being. Physiotherapists have used water for many years to assist with the rehabilitation of injuries and other medical conditions. Water-based exercise may include swimming, aqua aerobics, aqua circuit training, hydrotherapy, water walking and other variations of exercise in a water-based environment.

Exercising in water creates a very different physical experience for the body than exercising on land. This is because water has its own unique physical properties that will affect the body. These properties not only have an effect on the body systems, but also on how the body moves and the potential training benefits that can be obtained. Buoyancy and floatation offer support for the body and enable it to move more easily and without restriction. For example, a client who is overweight or who has restricted movement will be supported by the water and the improved movement and weightlessness they experience can feel liberating. In addition, the massaging effect of water will improve circulation and can assist relaxation and reduce muscular tension. There are also potentially more opportunities for social-isation in a water-based environment. The body is covered, so any potential self-consciousness is likely to be reduced. There is also the opportunity to develop sessions where participants work together in pairs or groups, which can build relationships and social networks.

Blue gyms are a network of organisations that deliver activities that are water-based or based near water. Activities may include wind surfing, water-skiing, sailing and a host of other activities based near or in water. For more information, visit www.bluegym.org.uk.

Community-based settings

Delivering programmes in different community settings (church halls, community centres, youth clubs, homes for the elderly, etc.) provides more opportunities for more people to be more active, without making the journey to a leisure club. Exercise and activity sessions delivered in the community can attract people who would not join a health and a leisure club, thus, making activity and exercise more accessible.

Community-based programmes may feel like a more relaxed setting. People may feel 'safer' and more confident to exercise alongside people they know and/or with others who may have the same experiences (e.g. a mental health condition). Being with people, who share similar experiences can reduce feelings of isolation, provide a support network and promote integration.

Hospital settings/secure units

For clients who are hospitalised this will be the primary setting of any intervention, including activity and exercise, for the duration of their hospitalisation. Activity programmes can be delivered both indoors and outdoors and may include gardening, walking, tai chi, chair-based exercise, dynamic or static relaxation, etc.

The benefits of working in this setting is that the exercise professional will have access to other health professionals who have a more detailed knowledge of the client and their specific needs. This offers the potential for a more collaborative working approach to promote the client's recovery.

TYPES OF EXERCISE INTERVENTION

All forms of exercise including the gym, classes, aqua, yoga and Pilates are suitable, although the content, length and intensity may need adjusting. Segregated classes (i.e. classes only for those with mental health conditions) are neither necessary nor helpful, as they may increase the feelings of being abnormal and not fit for society (exclusion).

To plan and deliver any form of exercise, the exercise professional must be qualified for that specific practical discipline (see Table 9.2). The old National Qualification Framework (NQF) is in the process of being replaced by the Qualification Curriculum Framework (QCF). Many of the existing qualifications that were developed prior to 2010 will continue to form part of that framework. The aim of the framework is to enable recognition of prior learning, so that specific areas of knowledge (anatomy and physiology, health and safety, etc.) will not have to be repeated to achieve additional qualifications.

Table 9.2	Different sessions and related qualifications		
Exercise disciplines	**Components of fitness trained**		**Related qualification**
	Advantages	*Disadvantages*	
Walking	• CV and endurance • Low impact • Accessible for most • Biophilia and other outdoor effects	• Safety may be an issue in some environments • Weather	Level 3 Walking Level 3 Outdoor Fitness Level 3 Training in Different Environments (TIDE)
Aqua	• All components trained • Fun, social, body is covered • Water properties therapeutic	• Non-swimmers • Persons with water phobias or other phobias (spread infection, etc.)	Level 2 Exercise in Water
Pilates	• Posture and core stability • Relaxing • Mobility and flexibility • Correct breathing	• No CV benefits • Some positions may be too challenging and need adaptation	Level 3 Pilates Matwork
Yoga	• Flexibility, mobility, balance, strength and endurance • Correct breathing and posture • Promotes relaxation and spiritual well-being	• Limited CV benefits • Some positions too challenging and need adaptation	Level 3 Yoga
Chair-based	• Mobility, maintenance of range of motion • Some strength benefits	• No CV benefits • Primarily aimed at frail elderly or very low fitness	Level 2 Chair-based exercise
Circuits	• Cardiovascular, strength and endurance	• Limited flexibility training unless specific activities included • May be seen as boot camp style – intimidating for some	Level 2 Circuit Training
Exercise to Music	• Cardiovascular, strength and endurance	• Coordination and motor skills challenged • Music and group exercise or studio environment may be intimidating	Level 2 Exercise to Music
Gym-based	• Cardiovascular, strength and endurance	• Limited flexibility training unless specific activities included • Machines can be intimidating • Gym environment can be intimidating/boring for some	Level 2 Gym Instructor

SESSION-PLANNING CONSIDERATIONS

Before planning the session there are a number of factors to take into account, from health and fitness status to body image.

Work capacity

Someone with a mental health condition is likely to have a low physical work capacity and possibly reduced movement ability, so planning an hour-long, intense session may be too optimistic in the early stages. For some an extended warm-up may be enough while others may manage only a warm-up and cool down. A main activity may not be introduced until a few weeks into the programme and should increase in duration rather than intensity in the first few months. An overall session time of 40 minutes is recommended as this will allow for a range of fitness and focus states. Motivation and self-esteem may be very low so any exercise programme must consider this and help with building a sense of achievement by incorporating easy-to-master exercises and intensities.

Clothing

Be flexible with regard to clothing and footwear, the person may not have anything else to wear so as long as it is clean and decent and shoes are stable and supportive, allow it. Suggest baggy comfortable clothing in the early stages to help ease body image problems and, if recommending classes, choose those attended by similar clients where possible.

Choreography

Avoid any high intensity, high impact or complex choreography with newcomers and have a range of contingency plans. Floor work may not be suitable as the lack of eye contact can cause discomfort in individuals and it is harder to monitor reactions.

EXERCISE CHOICE AND CONTRAINDICATIONS

There is no definitive list of exercises that work with mental health conditions. The physical ability and mental state of the individual will determine what they are capable of, and they may have firm goals or ideas about the type of exercise they want to do, which must be taken into account. Conversely, they may be unconcerned with the type of exercise and just go along with whatever you provide.

Find out about any exercise history of an individual – they may have been active before the onset of the condition and have a preferred activity in which they have a good level of ability and skill.

SESSION STRUCTURE

The traditional session structure is still appropriate for sessions with participants with mental health conditions. There should be a warm-up before the main session and a cool down after the main session (see Table 9.3). However, due to the nature of mental health conditions and the side effects of medication this structure may differ slightly. For example, the whole session may be just an extended warm-up and cool down with no main component or there may be more rest periods in the main component to allow recovery or to keep participants calm.

The intensity, content and exercises selected for the main session are determined by the client's goals and abilities.

Table 9.3	Session structure	
Warm-up	**Main workout**	**Cool down**
• Mobility and pulse raising • Appropriate pre-stretching exercises • Re-warming activities	Depending on the type of programme, may include: • Cardiovascular component: walking, aqua, ETM, step, CV machines, circuits and/or • Muscular fitness exercises: Body weight, aqua, resistance machines, bands, hand weights, free weights or • Yoga- and Pilates-based exercises • Chair-based work • Static and dynamic relaxation or tai chi	• Pulse lowering • Stretching (developmental and/or maintenance stretching as appropriate) • Relaxation

The warm-up

The warm-up is a very important part of a session as it is designed to prepare the body and mind for the main activity by providing a smooth transition from the resting state to the exercising state. Heart rate and blood flow to working muscles increase in a progressive manner, and the muscles, tendons, ligaments and joints used in the main activity are warmed up to help prevent injury or discomfort. To achieve this, the warm-up should incorporate pulse-raising, mobility and appropriate preparatory stretches.

The length of the warm-up will depend on the fitness level of the client and the overall length of the workout, but current guidelines (BACR, ACSM) recommend a minimum of 10 minutes and up to 15–20 minutes for longer sessions. It should increase very gradually in intensity and complexity to allow the body to adapt to the, possibly unaccustomed, increase in effort. An RPE of 2–3 on the modified scale is recommended.

• Consider chair-based moves initially for very unfit individuals, as the warm-up may be enough to provide an overload.
• Mix pulse-raising with mobility to create a mini-interval effect as this will maximise the effectiveness and avoid early fatigue. This will also foster a sense of achievement as they will be able to exercise for longer than they believed possible.
• There may be mobility issues for some so pre-stretching may need to be kept to a minimum and mixed with pulse-raising moves between each stretch to maintain warmth. Dynamic stretching may be more suitable, ensuring that moves are slow and controlled.

Main activity

The length of the main activity may vary from nothing in early stages to 30–40 minutes in later weeks. Cardiovascular work is important to encourage utilisation of fat stores and, initially, duration is more important than intensity to promote adherence. High intensity may be effective for fat burning but is likely to be uncomfortable and put the individual off.

As fitness levels are likely to be low, an interval approach may be necessary at first. Shorter bursts of cardio mixed with resistance work will help to keep the intensity raised and have the added benefits of improving muscle condition and helping to raise metabolic rate.

As fitness and exercise tolerance improves the cardio intervals can lengthen until the full 30 or 40 minutes is manageable. Once this stage is reached the individual may find that too long on one machine is boring (for a gym-based session) so using two or three machines or doing two blocks of cardio with some resistance in between may avoid this. An intensity of 4–6 on the RPE scale is recommended, however, always be guided by the client and encourage them to work within their comfort zone.

Cool down

Regardless of the intensity of the main activity a cool down is still an important part of the session. Any form of exertion causes blood supply to move to the working muscles and when exercise or exertion ceases it needs to be shunted back to the heart. While the intensity of the workout may not have been vigorous, it is likely to have been above normal levels so an effective cool down is important.

Keeping movement continuous while reducing the range and intensity of movement is advisable as if vigorous exercise is stopped abruptly there may be a reduced blood return to the heart, leading to a drop in cardiac output and blood pressure. The individual may feel dizzy, light-headed or weak and may experience an irregular heartbeat or sudden shortness of breath. Cramp may also occur. This is more common in individuals with existing cardiovascular disease or risk factors and in those with weakened systems.

Continuous movement, gradually decreasing in range and intensity, can be interspersed with abdominal and pelvic floor work before adding post-workout stretches. Maintenance or develop-mental stretches can be included as appro-priate for the individual and the 'try again' approach where a stretch is held for a shorter time but repeated two or three times to encourage flexibility may be useful.

It can be useful to explain that individuals will know when they are have cooled down sufficiently because they will feel less hot, their breathing will be back to normal, their heart rate is within 10–15bpm of normal and they are starting to 'dry off'.

The length of the cool down will reflect the overall session time, however, it is recommended that it is at least 10 minutes long for unfit clients to avoid arrhythmias (a side effect of some medication).

Relaxation

Following an appropriate cool down, a few minutes of relaxation may be beneficial for clients with hypertension or back pain and most individuals will feel the benefits of some quiet time. Learning basic relaxation techniques can help the person to cope with stress and anxiety and reduce the effects of these states on both the mind and body.

From simple breathing exercises to more advanced active muscle relaxation and tai chi style exercises, there are many forms of relaxation, so it is worth researching different techniques to find a method that best suits the individual or group.

Seated options including those that use the Laura Mitchell Method (extend and release method of active muscular relaxation) may be preferable to lying down and can be very effective. To download a leaflet about the Mitchell Method, visit www.acpwh.org.uk/docs/RelaxationLeaflet.pdf.

Following any form of relaxation it is essential to include some revitalising moves to ensure your client or group is fully awake and ready to return to normal activity.

SESSION DELIVERY
TEACHING AND DELIVERY METHODS

Instructing exercise to an individual or group with mental health conditions can be a challenge and will probably take you out of your teaching comfort zone and bring forth skills you did not know you had. This is not because these clients are difficult, but rather that they are often demotivated and lack the ability, meaning your competence in 'regressing' exercises will be important. Additionally, they may be vulnerable adults who may have experienced abuse or discrimination and are possibly feeling some shame or embarrassment about their condition.

It is the instructor's responsibility to ensure that the session goes well and this includes planning appropriate exercises or activities for the ability and condition of individuals. It is important to 'expect the unexpected' and be ready for anything. Consider teaching style – while there is no need to be patronising or talk down to people, it may cause confidence problems if the teaching style is very bouncy or forceful, and may even

trigger a confrontation out of uneasiness. It is best to adopt a reassuring, friendly and calm style while remaining professional to alleviate any nervousness the individual may be feeling.

At this point, building regularity is more important than becoming fitter, so an environment that feels welcoming and secure is more likely to bring people back on a regular basis. Keep feedback positive and encouraging and minimise 'correction' as it may be seem to highlight their perceived inability.

GYM INDUCTIONS AND SESSIONS
Equipment

The induction process may need to be split over several visits to allow the individual to become familiar with the machines and techniques, and process the information given. Shorter, more manageable sessions in the early weeks will help to avoid confusion or any sense of failure that may arise from being unfamiliar with the equipment and/or environment. Choose the equipment carefully; simple machines instead of complicated free weight exercises will foster a sense of achievement. You can bring in the complicated machines as self-efficacy and fitness develop.

Length

Sessions may need to vary in length. When you start out, a warm-up may be as much as the person can do, later a 30-minute session (or even shorter) may be enough and eventually a full hour may be achieved. This will vary from person to person and day to day and may be affected by changes in medication. Always be led by the individual – they may not look fatigued, but there may be emotional issues that mean they want to leave suddenly, often without explanation. If this should happen, thank them for coming and say you will see them at the next scheduled session. Never insist they stay or make them complete a cool down – sometimes people just need to go immediately.

If they do not want to continue to exercise but are happy to stay, use the time to discuss progress, set new goals or have a chat over a coffee!

GROUP EXERCISE CLASSES

Working with a group of people with a range of conditions is normal in exercise referral and this can cause problems with intensity. The type of class may need to be considered to ensure a positive experience is the outcome – circuits are often ideal while aerobics may be too complicated unless adapted. Again, your plans for any session will depend on the ability and fitness levels of the group and even the best-laid plans can go horribly wrong.

EXERCISE TO MUSIC

Your cues may need to be adapted for this client group as longer lead-in times and simpler signals will help them to follow the moves. Your demonstrations must be clear and slow to enable the group to follow the routine. The use of simple, clear teaching points and instructions will help to keep everyone on track. Think about voice tone as well, remain positive and avoid shouting, as it can be distressing.

Choreography should be simple and build up gradually. Use repetition to reinforce the moves. Music may need to be slower than usual to allow for lower fitness and skill levels.

The use of praise as well as correction is important, and if some of the moves are a bit iffy, so what – keep the praise going and ensure your movements are good and in time good technique will start to happen. Moving round to observe may unsettle the group so ensure you do keep an eye on everyone and reinforce technique with a few well-chosen words. Please note that the use of touch may be very unwelcome, particularly if there is a history of abuse, so avoid this as much as possible.

Alternatives are essential; experience has shown that if it can go wrong it will, so have several contingency plans just in case. There may be times when nothing works so be prepared to switch to a relaxation session or even finish early if necessary.

CIRCUITS

The benefit of circuits is that they are easy to run with a group of mixed ability participants and adaptations can be planned in advance to ensure everyone has an appropriate workout.

The circuit emphasis can be cardiovascular, muscular strength and endurance (MSE), functional or sporty and the intensity can be low, moderate and high across the same group. It may be better to keep intensity low to moderate for any referred session to avoid the risk of client's overdoing it, since they might feel the need to 'prove' their ability. Simple exercises using very basic equipment will make it easy to monitor and control the session.

Whatever the type of session and whoever the clients are, the most important qualities you can demonstrate as an instructor are those of quiet confidence, friendliness and being non-judgemental.

An overview of teaching methods is shown in table 9.4.

Table 9.4	Teaching methods	
Method	**When used**	**Issues and considerations**
Demonstration	• To show an exercise • To demonstrate correct alignment and technique	• The fitness professional must be able to demonstrate accurately. • Physical or intellectual disability (visual, hearing, learning, physical) may require other methods to be used.
Question and answer	• To ask a client what they are experiencing (thinking or feeling) e.g. where they feel a stretch or how hard an activity is perceived to be (RPE)	• The fitness professional must ask appropriate questions to elicit accurate information from the client. • They must also be able to respond to the answer the client provides, e.g. if the client answers that they find an exercise difficult or uncomfortable.
Explanation and instruction	• To explain and educate on the benefits and effects of doing a particular exercise, e.g. 'You should feel this here.'	• The fitness professional must speak clearly and audibly and use appropriate and accessible language. • They must also check understanding through questioning.
Adaptation, progression and regression	• To enable clients to work at a level that is appropriate for them	• The fitness professional must be aware of the principles of training (frequency, intensity, time and type) and be able to apply these to a range of contexts to ensure activities and exercises are suitable. • They must also be aware of the impact of the principles that vary intensity (repetitions, rate, resistance, rest, range of motion) and be able to adapt exercises using these variables.

MONITORING INTENSITY

The most accessible methods of monitoring intensity are the talk test and RPE scales.

Talk test

Working to a level where one can breathe comfortably, rhythmically and hold a conversation while exercising is suggested to indicate an appropriate intensity (see Table 9.5). Although the method is very simplistic and quite subjective, it can serve as a useful guide to indicate how hard someone may be working. It would not be appropriate for persons who choose not to speak.

Table 9.5	Talk test	
Intensity level	**Talk test response while exercising**	**Action**
Too high	If one or only a few words can be spoken	Lower the intensity to a manageable level
Too low	If a number of sentences can be spoken too comfortably	Increase the intensity
Appropriate	If a mild breathlessness is apparent at the end of speaking a couple of sentences	Maintain this level of intensity

Table 9.6	The Borg 6–20 RPE scale and CR10 scale						
6–20 RPE		**Min HR**	**Mean HR**	**Max HR**	**Comments**	**Modified RPE/CR10**	
No exertion at all	6	69	77	91		Nothing at all	0
Extremely light	7	76	85	101	Warm-up/ cool down zone	Very, very weak	0.5
	8	83	93	111			
Very light	9	89	101	122		Very weak	1
	10	96	110	132		Weak	2
Light	11	103	118	142		Moderate	3
	12	110	126	153		Somewhat strong	4
Somewhat hard	13	116	135	163	Aerobic zone		5
	14	123	143	173		Strong	6
Hard (heavy)	15	130	151	184		Very strong	7
	16	137	159	194			8
Very hard	17	143	168	204			9
	18	150	176	215	Intervals – anaerobic zone		
Extremely hard	19	157	184	225		Very, very strong	10
Max exertion	20	164	193	235			

The Rating of Perceived Exertion (RPE)

The RPE scale is used to quantify the subjective intensity of exercise. The participant is encouraged to focus on the sensations of physical exertion, such as feelings of breathlessness, strain and fatigue in muscles, and then to rate his or her overall feelings of exertion using the scale. The more experienced a client becomes at detecting and rating sensations, the more closely the ratings correlate with the exercise intensity. However, clients with anxiety disorders may over-estimate the sensations, because these feel like symptoms of their conditions.

SP

Research has shown that individuals can perceive how hard they are working quite accurately on a scale (Borg, 1967, 1982). The Rating of Perceived Exertion (RPE) scale runs from 6 to 20 and is supposed to reflect heart rates ranging from 60–200bpm. The CR10 scale runs from 0–10. Instructors must be aware that it takes time and practice to become proficient at predicting exertion rates.

It is recommended that for aerobic work, intensity should remain somewhere between 11 and 16 on the RPE scale (between 3 and 7 on the CR10 scale).

PROGRESSION, REGRESSION AND ADAPTATION OF EXERCISES

The frequency, intensity, duration and type of exercise will need to correspond to the needs of the individual, including:

- the fitness level of the individual;
- the medical condition/s with which they have been referred;
- the effects of any medication on the exercise response; and
- any other specific lifestyle considerations (work, etc.)

Previously inactive people will generally have to work at a lower intensity and possibly for shorter durations. They may also have lower levels of body awareness, lower levels of fitness and skill, and their exercise technique may demand more careful attention and supervision from the exercise professional (teaching, observation, correction) to enable safe performance. However, it is important to remember that enjoyment of the session is paramount so if a participant is doing an exercise incorrectly, but not unsafely, it may not be appropriate to attempt corrections more than once or twice.

There are specific variants that can be altered to change and adapt the intensity of specific exercises. These are shown in table 9.7.

When progressing or regressing, one single variable should be added (or removed) at a time.

Table 9.7	Variables for regression and progression	
Variable	**Regression**	**Progression**
Repetitions	Do less	Do more
Range of motion	Smaller	Larger
Resistance	Lighter Remove weight Use body weight Use shorter levers	Heavier Add weight Use weights or bands Lengthen levers
Rate	Slow it down	Increase the pace
Rest	Allow more rests Use an interval or fartlek approach with longer rests and shorter work time Use fewer working sets of the same exercise or fewer exercises	Less rests Use a continuous approach or use an interval or fartlek approach with shorter rests and longer work time Use more sets of the same exercise or more exercises

When building up a programme it would not be progressive suddenly to increase a number of variables at the same time. This may create overwork, rather than the desired overload.

OBSERVATION AND MONITORING

While any experienced instructor will be used to observing exercise technique and giving feedback, there is another reason for keen observational skills when working with clients with mental health problems. Individuals are often reluctant to say that they feel unwell, are finding the activity too hard or easy, if they feel unable to cope with new situations, or want to leave, and they may suddenly display a change in behaviour to get round this.

This change can manifest in a number of ways, usually physically or emotionally and some of the more commons signs are shown in figure 9.1.

These signs may mean the individual is simply feeling tired or bored or they may be on the verge of a panic attack so it is important to keep monitoring the individual or group and remain on the lookout for any of these changes. If observed, consider the likely cause; if it is tiredness or boredom, change the activity – offer to show a new exercise you think

they may enjoy, bring the group together in a circuit and do some static work or break up an aerobic routine with some MSE work.

Alternatively, you can ask if they want to leave or sit down for a while. Early intervention may avoid an escalation of emotion or behaviour into an uncontrollable event (see Chapter 7, page 146).

SUMMARY POINTS

You should now be able to:

- List some of the things that need to be considered prior to planning a session.
- Describe the advantages and disadvantages of working in different environments and settings.
- Describe the main components of a safe session structure.
- State the advantages and disadvantages of different types of sessions.
- Discuss the merits of different session types for working with specific conditions with consideration to comorbidities/medications.
- Describe methods for monitoring intensity.
- Recognise methods for progressing and regressing different activities.

Changes in	Signs of	Becoming
• Voice tone • Posture • Facial expression • Body language • Movement speed or quality • Speech patterns • Breathing rate or depth • Eye contact • Coordination	• Paranoia • Anger • Misunderstanding • Tearfulness • Shame or embarrassment • Withdrawal or attention seeking • Attachment or dismissal	• Louder or quieter • Rude • Confrontational or argumentative • Impatient or frustrated • Apologetic • Competitive

Figure 9.1 Signs of distress

APPENDICES

APPENDIX 1: LEGISLATION AND ORGANISATIONS

LEGISLATION

The Mental Capacity Act (2005)
Legislation that outlines the legal provisions for persons who lack capacity.

www.legislation.gov.uk/ukpga/2005/9/contents

The Mental Health Act (MHA, 1983, 2007)
Legislation that sets out the criteria that must be met before compulsory action is taken, to ensure people with mental disorders get the care and treatment they need for their own health or safety, or for the protection of other people (see appendix 5, page 181).

www.dh.gov.uk/en/Publicationsandstatistics/Legislation

The Mental Health Action Plan (2006/2009) – Wales
Outlines 12 actions for mental health services across Wales.

wales.gov.uk/publications

The Disability Discrimination Act (DDA)
Promotes civil rights for disabled people and protects disabled people from discrimination.

www.direct.gov.uk/disability

'A person has a disability for the purposes of this Act if he has a physical or mental impairment which has a substantial and long-term adverse effect on his ability to carry out normal day-to-day activities.'

www.opsi.gov.uk/acts/acts1995/ukpga_19950050_en_2#pt1-l1g1

Equality Act 2010
This Act simplifies discrimination legislation and covers discrimination relating to a range of individuals including but not limited to; disability, age, race, culture, religious beliefs, sexual orientation, gender, pregnant, post natal and breastfeeding women. It also covers issues relating to victimisation and harassment.

The Equality Act 2010 replaced most of the Disability Discrimination Act (DDA), however the Disability Equality Duty (DED) in the DDA is still in force. Disability Equality Duty applies to public sector organisations such as hospitals, educational establishments, NHS, police and government. For more information on DED visit: www.direct.gov.uk/en/DisabledPeople/RightsAndObligations/DisabilityRights/DG_10038105. For both Acts, the definition of disability is as follows:

'A person has a disability for the purposes of this Act if he has a physical or mental impairment which has a substantial and long-term effect on the ability to carry out normal day-to-day activities'.

www.equalities.gov.uk/equality_act_2010

ORGANISATIONS

National Institute for Health and Clinical Excellence (NICE)

NICE is an independent organisation responsible for providing national clinical guidance (published and in development) on promoting good health and preventing and treating ill health.

www.nice.org.uk

Department of Health (DoH)

Government department responsible for public health issues.

www.dh.gov.uk

Care Quality Commission (CQC)

An independent regulator of health and social care in England. It regulates care provided by the NHS, local authorities, private companies and voluntary organisations. It protects the interests of people whose rights are restricted under the MHA and ensures better service is provided.

www.cqc.org.uk

The Scottish Government

The devolved government for Scotland is responsible for issues of concern to the population of Scotland, including health and mental health services. The Chief Medical Officer is the principal medical adviser and has direct involvement in health policy for Scotland, including improving the mental and physical well-being of people in Scotland.

www.scotland.gov.uk

Northern Ireland Assembly

The Northern Ireland Assembly is the devolved legislature for Northern Ireland with the responsibility for passing laws on transferred matters, including mental and physical health.

www.northernireland.gov.uk/index.htm

Fitness Wales

Fitness Wales is a charitable organisation, established over 40 years ago as the governing body for exercise and fitness in Wales with sup- port and funding from the Sports Council of Wales. Fitness Wales are one of the first organisations to receive approval from SkillsActive to deliver training for the Level 4 Physical Activity for Persons with Mental Health Conditions national occupational standards.

www.fitnesswales.co.uk

SkillsActive

SkillsActive is the sector skills council representing the sport and active leisure sector. It develops qualification frameworks and sets the national occupational standards to ensure the sector meets specific needs. SkillsActive endorses training courses available through its Endorsement Committee, Technical Expert Group (TEG) and the Register of Exercise Professionals (REPs).

www.skillsactive.com

The Register of Exercise Professionals (REPs)

REPs was set up with support from SkillsActive to help safeguard the interests of people using the services of exercise and fitness instructors, teachers and trainers. REPs provides occupational descriptors for specific working roles within the fitness industry. It also provides a code of practice that outlines the appropriate ethical working requirements for the sector.

The Medical Defence Union and Medical Protection Society acknowledge REPs as a professional body, recognised by the Department of Health. GPs can refer clients to advanced fitness instructors (level 3) with qualifications and experience of working with special/referred populations.

www.exerciseregister.org

Fitness Industry Association (FIA) Code of Practice

The FIA has developed a code of practice that is designed to ensure that health and fitness operators maintain a basic level of practice to ensure the safety and well-being of their customers. By complying with the standards of the code the industry can raise the level of operation throughout all FIA facilities.

www.fia.org.uk/about-us/FIA-Code-of-Practice.html

The UK Quality Scheme for Sport and Leisure (QUEST)

QUEST aims to define industry standards and good practice through encouraging ongoing development and delivery within a customer-focused management framework.

www.questnbs.info

Inclusive Fitness Initiative (IFI)

The IFI supports leisure facility operators to become more inclusive, catering for the needs of disabled and non-disabled people to raise physical activity participation levels. The IFI also operate a accreditation scheme called the IFI Mark, which is a quality mark for fitness facilities based upon the principles of the IFI.

www.inclusivefitness.org

Mental Health Foundation (MHF)

A charity that supports and campaigns for persons with mental health conditions.

www.mentalhealth.org.uk

Depression Alliance UK

A charity that supports people with depression.

www.depressionalliance.org

Journeys

The Depression Alliance in Wales was relaunched as Journeys. This organisation provides information, practical resources, services and training that promote the development of skills and strategies to help people find their own route to recovery.

www.journeysonline.org.uk

Rethink

A national charity founded over 30 years ago that provides support and help to give a voice to those affected by severe and enduring mental illness – schizophrenia, schizoaffective disorder and bipolar disorder.

www.rethink.org

Mind

A mental health charity supporting persons with mental health conditions in England and Wales. It campaigns to influence change and improve services, legislation, legal rights and acceptance for persons with mental health conditions.

www.mind.org.uk

Hafal

A leading charity in Wales supporting people with serious mental illness and their carers.

www.hafal.org

The Scottish Association for Mental Health (SAMH)

SAMH is the leading mental health charity in Scotland and promotes awareness of mental health issues and campaigns for the development of legislation and policies relating to mental health issues. SAMH support a range of initiatives and programmes that address issues such as stigma, bullying and suicide prevention in Scotland.

www.samh.org.uk

Northern Ireland Association for Mental Health (NIAMH)

NIAMH is the oldest mental health organisation in Northern Ireland and aims to support individuals with mental health issues and promote mental well-being throughout society. It is involved with research and policy development and promotes well-being in businesses as well as individuals.

www.niamhwellbeing.org

The Royal College of Psychiatrists

The professional and educational body for psychiatrists in the United Kingdom. Their three key aims are to:

- Set standards and promote excellence in psychiatry and mental healthcare
- Lead, represent and support psychiatrists
- Work with service users, carers and their organisations

For further information see www.rcpsych.ac.uk.

APPENDIX 2: OTHER USEFUL WEBSITES

All Wales Mental Health Promotion Network: www.publicmentalhealth.org

Alcoholics Anonymous: www.alcoholics-anonymous.org.uk

The Association for Postnatal Illness (APNI): Helpline: 020 7386 0868 (10am–2pm Mon, Weds and Fri and 10am–5pm, Tues and Thurs); www.apni.org

Aware – Helping to defeat depression (information and support to people affected by depression in Ireland and Northern Ireland): Helpline 00 353 1 90 303 302; Tel. 00 353 1 661 7211; www.aware.ie

The British Association for Counselling and Psychotherapy (BACP): www.bacp.co.uk

Centre for Mental Health: www.centreformentalhealth.org.uk/index.aspx

Change 4 Life: www.nhs.uk/Change4life

Change 4 Life Cymru: www.wales.gov.uk/hcwsubsite healthchallenge/individuals/change

Cruse Bereavement Care:
www.crusebereavementcare.org.uk/About Grief.html

Depression UK: www.depressionuk.org; Email info@depressionuk.org

Drinkaware (alcohol help/awareness): www.drinkaware.co.uk

Food and Mood Project Survey: www.news.bbc.co.uk/2/hi/health/2264529.stm

FRANK (drugs help/awareness): www.talktofrank.com

Living Life to the Full (Cognitive Behavioural Therapy online course): www.livinglifetothefull.com

MDF The Bipolar Organisation Cymru: Tel. 08456 340 540; www.mdf.org.uk

Mental Health Foundation (MHF): www.mentalhealth.org.uk/about-us

Narcolepsy Association UK: www.narcolepsy.org.uk

National Association for Premenstrual Syndrome: Phone/fax. 0870 777 2178; www.pms.org.uk

National Sleep Foundation: www.sleepfoundation.org

Overcoming Anorexia: www.overcominganorexiaonline.com

Overcoming Bulimia: www.overcomingbulimiaonline.com

National Institute of Mental Health (NIMH): www.nimh.nih.gov

Physical Activity and Nutrition Networks: www.physicalactivityandnutritionwales.org.uk

Relate (counselling, therapy, sex education): www.relate.org.uk

Samaritans: www.samaritans.org

SANE (mental health charity): Tel. 0845 767 8000; www.sane.org.uk

The Sleep Council: www.sleepcouncil.org.uk

Smoking cessation (various): www.quitsmoking.com

SmokeFree: www.smokefree.nhs.uk

Time to Change. A social movement in England to challenge stigma attached to mental health: www.time-to-change.org.uk/home

Wales Mental Health Promotion: www.publicmentalhealth.org

Walking for Health: www.wfh.naturalengland.org.uk

YoungMinds (The voice for young people's mental health and well-being): Tel. 020 7336 8445; www.youngminds.org.uk

APPENDIX 3: MENTAL HEALTH SERVICES CARE PROVISION

Over 300 people in every 1000 experience mental health problems every year in Britain and of these 230 will visit a GP. From there, 102 people will be diagnosed as having a mental health problem and 24 will then be referred to a specialist psychiatric service with 6 becoming inpatients in psychiatric hospitals.

PRIMARY CARE

As the figures above show, initial care provision is usually within the primary care setting. The GP may offer medication, therapy or exercise on referral as treatment options, depending on the severity of the problem or availability of these options.

Exercise referral schemes are an option in the early stages of a condition or in the recovery phase for those who prefer to try a range of treatment options. Doctors and other health professionals can refer the patient for a fixed term of supervised activity and exercise within community facilities and there are opportunities for patients to be referred into such schemes when discharged from more formal treatment or care provision.

SECONDARY CARE

Outside the primary care setting, there are a variety of care options for people needing mental health services at all levels. This 'secondary care' falls broadly into three main categories:

1 Community-based care services
2 Clinical care services
3 Secure care services

Community-based care services

This is overseen by the community mental health team (CMHT). Within the CMHT there are designated roles to provide support and assistance to patients living in the community, and to ensure medication compliance. The team includes community psychiatric nurses (CPNs) who form part of the CMHT and work alongside psychiatrists, psychologists, counsellors, occupational therapists and social workers.

Key roles of the CMHT include crisis resolution and early intervention in psychosis, home treatment, recovery and outreach for harder to engage people. Patients may also have access to domiciliary care, such as meals on wheels and home help, and be referred to occupation therapy within larger units to provide structure and activity to help with recovery.

The crisis resolution team (CRT) may also be involved in care. The CRT is available to support adults experiencing a severe mental health crisis in the community without admission to a psychiatric unit, if appropriate. If the crisis is manageable in the community or at home, a crisis management plan involving treatment and support will be developed and put into place.

Community-based residential care is an option for some as independence can be maintained with appropriate supervision. This includes a range of options such as supported housing, providing a range of care from rehabilitation to activities of daily living, sheltered accommodation, hostels, respite homes and residential homes. There are also many homes and housing options run by charities and religious groups.

Clinical and secure care services

These include psychiatric units with intensive treatment wards and acute treatment wards, depending on the severity of the condition and the risk of harm.

Secure mental health services include high, medium and low secure services for adults with mental health disorders, including personality disorders, who are deemed to present a significant risk of harm to themselves and others, and medium and low secure hospitals. Most, but not all, will be convicted offenders and usually all will be detained under the Mental Health Act (see appendix 5, page 181). These include high security facilities such as Ashworth in Merseyside, Broadmoor in Berkshire and Rampton in Nottinghamshire, each part of an NHS Trust. Patients in high secure facilities are considered to present a serious and significant risk to the public and will be detained for a significant period for treatment. There are approximately 800 high secure places, or beds, in these facilities.

Medium secure services provide treatment over a shorter period of time, typically 2–5 years, for adults who are deemed to present a significant or serious danger to the public. Many will have been transferred from prison or directly from court (which is known as 'court disposal') and will have a history of offending. There are approximately 3,500 medium secure beds in total, of which around 35% are independently managed.

Low secure services are used to treat people who present a risk, to either themselves or others, or who are considered unsuitable for open mental health treatment settings. As with medium secure settings, patients may have been transferred from court or prison for inpatient treatment. The recommended maximum stay in low secure facilities is eight weeks and patients are either detained from the community or have been 'stepped down' from medium secure services.

Medium and low secure facilities are run by both NHS trusts and independent organisations with the majority of admissions (approximately 99%) to NHS facilities and the remainder to independent hospitals or facilities. Of all admissions, approximately 14–15% are formal admissions under the Mental Health Act.

Note: There are many other services available within the community. For full information download the MIND factsheet, Community based mental health and social care, available from: www.mind.org.uk/help/community_care/community-based_mental_health_and_social_care.

The Care Programme Approach (CPA)

The CPA was introduced in England in 1991 and Scotland in 1997 and is a patient-centred, confidential care and support plan for every person who is accepted into specialist mental health services. It is a means of coordinating community-based care and services to meet individual, cultural, linguistic and gender needs arising from a mental health problem. The CPA requires that health and social services:

- assess need;
- provide a written care plan;
- allocate a care coordinator (formerly known as the key worker) and
- review the plan regularly.

Ideally, people with a CPA should be able to access appropriate care or services at any time of the day or night and on any day of the year.

Terms used in forensic psychiatry

- **Legal competence** involves several categories and is determined by an assessment of the capacity to understand actions.
- **Testamentary capacity** refers to the capability to make, and understand the making of, a will and that capability is not distorted by a mental health disorder.
- **Fitness to plead** is where a jury decides if the defendant has the capacity to defend charges.
- **Mens rea**, or guilty mind, establishes whether a person is criminally responsible either by virtue of age (under 10s are deemed not to be criminally responsible), psychiatric illness or lack of criminal intent, where the action was accidental.
- **Automatism** covers disassociation between the action and the mind, for example, an act committed when sleepwalking or concussed.
- **Diminished responsibility** is where a specific 'abnormality of mind' substantially impairs mental function and responsibility and can allow a homicide charge to be reduced to manslaughter.

FORENSIC PSYCHIATRY

Working in forensic psychiatry involves working with individuals who have been convicted of a crime or who are awaiting trial and have a diagnosed mental health disorder. It is rare for someone with a mental health disorder to commit crimes of a violent nature, as most people with a severe mental health problem are more likely to harm themselves than another person.

APPENDIX 4: MENTAL HEALTH SERVICES KEY STAFF

There are many people that service users may meet during treatment.

GENERAL PRACTITIONER (GP)

The GP is often the first person involved in mental health treatment and is key in the identification of a condition and discussion of treatment options.

PSYCHIATRIST

A psychiatrist deals with both physical and psychological aspects of the condition and any necessary medication or pharmacological interventions. As a qualified medical doctor, the psychiatrist will have undertaken additional training in mental health conditions. Psychiatrists work in hospital, forensic and community settings and are usually the most senior member of the care team. Patients may encounter the consultant psychiatrist's assistant, the registrar, more often than the consultant.

PSYCHOLOGIST

A psychologist will look at the connection between thoughts and feelings and actions. There are two key types involved in mental health:

1 The **clinical psychologist** is concerned with the assessment and treatment of mental health conditions. They will help an individual identify, alleviate and manage the cause of their mental health problems. They offer treatment, including cognitive behavioural therapy (CBT) and psychotherapy.

2 The **counselling psychologist** will use a range of approaches and talking treatments through a collaborative relationship with the individual to empower and motivate them to make changes in their lives.

PSYCHOTHERAPIST

Psychotherapy may be a deeper and longer term form of counselling or talking therapy, which aims to help the individual understand why they feel and act or respond the way they do.

COUNSELLOR

Counsellors practice 'talking therapies' and provide opportunities to talk about thoughts and feelings and then help to identify coping strategies to enable a change in life patterns. Sessions may be individual-, family- or group-based.

CARE MANAGER

The care manager is not involved in direct care or service delivery, rather the role is focused on assessing social care needs and arranging delivery of care services for many different client groups within the local authority under the NHS and Community Care Act (1990). The care manager will work with the Community Mental Health Team (CMHT) when arranging services or care for individuals with mental health problems.

CARE COORDINATOR

Usually part of the CMHT, the care coordinator is a named point of contact for the individual with mental health problems. Formerly known as the key worker, they will monitor the CPA for the individual and provide ongoing support.

COMMUNITY MENTAL HEALTH/ PSYCHIATRIC NURSE (CMHN/CPN)

The role of the CPN is to support individuals with mental health conditions in the community. Individuals may have been discharged from a unit and part of the role of the CMHN is to support them and help avoid relapse or readmission into the psychiatric unit. They can also administer medication and injections.

APPROVED MENTAL HEALTH PROFESSIONAL (AMHP)

This is a relatively new role, created in November 2008. It replaces the approved social worker role and can now include other mental health personnel such as psychologists, occupational therapists and psychiatric nurses, if approved. All AMHPs have extensive training in the Mental Health Act and their key role is to assess individuals for detention under the act and make the necessary application. Each local authority or health board must ensure that AMHPs are available at all times in the event of emergency assessment and/or admission.

APPROVED SOCIAL WORKER (ASW)

The ASW traditionally played a significant role in supporting individuals with mental health conditions. Following the Mental Health Act 2007, the ASW role is replaced by the AMHP.

The occupational therapist (OT) works in all types of setting and helps individuals with mental health problems to learn, or relearn, the skills needed for daily life. They provide activities to promote skills in self-care, domestic, social and work areas together with individual counselling and group work activities in stress and anxiety management, assertiveness and anger management training.

COMMUNITY MENTAL HEALTH TEAM (CMHT)

The CMHT is made up of a range of mental health professionals who deliver mental health services in the community. Key personnel are the psychiatrist, counsellor/psychologist, CPN, AMHP, OT and care coordinator.

Health visitor

Qualified nurse with specialist mental health training who can offer support and advice about health and living issues and local services.

Social worker

A useful source of advice and information on practical issues such as finances, benefits and accommodation.

The nearest relative (NR)

Under the Mental Health Act, the patient's nearest relative (NR) has certain rights to protect the patient's interests. The NR is usually the person who is highest on the following list:

- Husband, wife or civil partner
- Partner (of either sex) who has lived with the patient for at least six months
- Son or daughter
- Father or mother
- Brother or sister

- Grandfather or grandmother
- Uncle or aunt
- Nephew or niece
- Has lived with the person for at least five years, but is not related

Crisis resolution team (CRT)

Crisis resolution teams treat people who are currently experiencing an acute and severe psychiatric crisis. Treatment will occur at a day care centre, the person's home, or in a crisis residential home or hostel. Without their involvement, the person would require hospital treatment. The CRT is responsible for planning aftercare once the crisis has ended, to prevent further episodes.

APPENDIX 5: THE MENTAL HEALTH ACT (MHA)

THE MENTAL HEALTH ACT (ENGLAND AND WALES) 1983

Note: There have been many amendments to the MHA 1983 which are included in the information below. For a full copy of the Act, visit the Department of Health website at: www.dh.gov.uk/en/Healthcare/Mentalhealth/Information ontheMentalHealthAct/index.htm or for the relevant information for Wales visit www.wales.nhs.uk/sites3/home.cfm?orgid=816.

The Mental Health Act exists to allow compulsory detention of an individual with a mental health condition for assessment and/or treatment where that detention or treatment is necessary for a) their own health and safety and b) the health and safety or protection of others. It

sets out the criteria that must be met before such compulsory measures can be made, together with protections and safeguards for patients. The Act is divided into parts, each with a number of sections and when a section is applied to a person it is often referred to as 'being sectioned'.

An instructor is only likely to encounter sections of the Act when working in secure or clinical facilities, at which time any relevant sections or implications will be explained as necessary.

PART 1: APPLICATION OF THE ACT

This sets out the terms of reference of 'mental disorder' as any disorder or disability of the mind. In particular it identifies that learning disability is not considered a mental disorder unless other additional behaviours are present.

PART 2: COMPULSORY ADMISSION TO HOSPITAL AND GUARDIANSHIP

Part 2 outlines the civil procedures to be followed for detention in hospital for either assessment or treatment of mental disorder. In order for detention to occur, a formal application must be made by either an approved mental health professional or the patient's nearest relative (see overleaf). For the application to be granted, two medical recommendations must be made by two qualified medical professionals, one approved for purpose under the Act. Part 2 also covers the procedures for application for guardianship under the Act.

There are many sections of the Act, and those more frequently used are summarised in the table overleaf.

Appendix 5.1 — Frequently used sections of the Mental Health Act

Section	Title	Procedure	Duration
2	Admission for assessment	Application made by AMHP, NR. Confirmed by two registered medical practitioners (RMP) that the patient has a mental disorder that warrants detention in hospital for assessment for at least a limited period AND that he/she should be detained in interests of his/her health and safety or the protection of others.	Up to 28 days
3	Admission for treatment	Application by NR (or AMHP if NR does not object, is displaced by county court or not reasonably practical to consult NR and confirmation by two RMPs that the patient has a mental disorder that makes it appropriate to receive treatment in hospital **AND** appropriate medical treatment is available **AND** it is necessary for his/her own safety or for protection of others to receive such treatment which cannot be provided unless detained under this section.	Up to 6 months, renewable for a further 6 months then 1 year at a time
4	Admission for assessment in cases of emergency	Application by AMHP or NR and confirmation by one RMP that it is of 'urgent necessity' for the patient to be admitted and detained under Section 2 **AND** waiting for a second RMP would cause 'undesirable delay'.	Up to 72 hours
5 (2)	Application in respect of patient already in hospital	A RMP in charge of an informal patient's treatment can detain a patient by reporting that an application for compulsory admission *ought to be made*.	Up to 72 hours
5 (4)		A nurse trained to work in mental illness can detain an informal patient who is already receiving treatment for mental disorder until an RMP arrives.	Up to 6 hours
135	Warrant to search for and remove patients	Issued to police officer and RMP/AMHP if cause to suspect a person has a mental disorder **AND** is being ill-treated or neglected or not under proper control **OR** lives alone and is unable to care for self.	Up to 72 hours
136	Mentally disordered persons found in public places	Police officer can remove a person to a place of safety (hospital or police station) if that person appears to be suffering from a mental disorder and is in immediate need of care or control.	Up to 72 hours

Part 3: Patients Concerned in Criminal Proceedings or under Sentence

Part 3 relates to the criminal justice system and outlines the powers of the court (crown and/or magistrates) to remand an accused person to hospital for treatment or report on their mental disorder. It also applies to the detention in hospital for treatment of a person convicted of an offence. Key sections are detailed in the table below.

Appendix 5.2	Key sections of Part 3 of the Mental Health Act		
Section	**Title**	**Procedure**	**Duration**
35	Remand to hospital for report on accused's mental condition	Remanded to hospital on evidence from a registered medical practitioner (RMP) that there is reason to suspect that he/she is suffering from an mental disorder AND It would be impracticable for a report on his/her mental condition to be made if he/she were remanded on bail.	Up to 28 days, renewable for further periods of 28 days up to a maximum of 12 weeks in total.
36	Remand to hospital for treatment	Remanded to hospital for treatment on evidence from two RMPs that he/she is suffering from a mental disorder that makes detention for treatment appropriate and that appropriate treatment is available.	Up to 28 days, renewable for further periods of 28 days up to a maximum of 12 weeks in total.
37	Hospital order	Detention in hospital of a convicted offender on evidence from two RMPs that the offender has a mental disorder that makes detention for medical treatment appropriate and that appropriate medical treatment is available and that a hospital order is the most suitable option.	
38	Interim hospital order	As above on evidence from two RMPs that a convicted offender has a mental disorder and there is reason to suppose it is appropriate for the order to be made.	
41	Power of higher courts to restrict discharge from hospital	Imposed in addition to section 37 if it is necessary to protect public from 'serious harm' and a least one of the RMPs who recommended section 37 gave evidence orally. Made by Crown Court.	No set duration, discharge by application.
47	Transfer to hospital from prison	Ordered by the Secretary of State for Justice if satisfied by evidence from two RMPs that an offender has a mental disorder that makes detention for medical treatment appropriate and that appropriate medical treatment is available.	Up to 6 months, renewable for a further 6 months then one year at a time.

Part 4: Consent to Treatment

There are two main parts to this section of the MHA; the first relates to treatments for formal patients and states that treatment can be given without consent unless the MHA or DoH regulations specify otherwise. The second part covers supervised community treatment (SCT) for a period of six months following the end of formal detention. The sections in part 4 of the MHA are complicated and it is recommended that you read the MHA if you wish to know more.

Admissions

Figures relating to the application of the MHA in 2002/2 show that 55 per cent of admissions (13,800) related to Section 2, 35 per cent (8,500) were under section 3 and 8 per cent (1,800) were under section 4. Court and prison disposals under Part 3 of the MHA were 5 per cent of admissions.

THE MENTAL HEALTH (CARE AND TREATMENT) SCOTLAND ACT 2003

The Mental Health (Care and Treatment) Scotland Act 2003 covers the compulsory care and treatment of people with mental health disorders. In order to be detained, the person must be suffering from a mental health disorder, including mental illness, dementia, personality disorder or learning disability, that significantly impairs their decision making regarding the treatment of their condition and where non-detention would put their health, safety or welfare and the health, safety or welfare of others at significant risk.

The Act is independently monitored and applies to prisoners and those awaiting trial as well. It has many orders (or sections hence the term 'being sectioned') each referring to a particular aspect of detention, treatment or assessment and a link to the legislation is given below.

For an overview of the Mental Health (C&T) Scotland Act 2003 visit www.opsi.gov.uk/legislation/scotland/acts2003/asp_20030013_en_1(Scotland) and for an overview of mental health services in Scotland visit: www.audit-scotland.gov.uk/docs/health/2009/nr_090514_mental_health.pdf.

Any particular aspects of the Act that relate to an environment in which you are working will be explained to you, however, as an overview, the Mental Health (Care and Treatment) Scotland Act 2003 can be summarised as follows:

- Compulsory care and treatment is to be used only as a last resort and must be linked the patient's care plan.
- It allows for treatment without consent in the community (a less restrictive alternative to hospital detention).
- It is a new independent tribunal, replacing the role of the sheriff court, to consider compulsory measures.
- Aims to clarify and strengthen the rights of carers.
- Reforms the system for dealing with mentally disordered offenders, including new arrangements for the discharge of restricted patients.

A patient must have the following requirements for compulsory detention under the Mental Health (C&T) Scotland Act 2003:

- A mental disorder which significantly impairs decision-making ability with respect to medical treatment.

Admission is necessary for:

- patient's health or safety;

and/or

- the protection of others.

Emergency detention

Any fully registered medical practitioner may grant a certificate authorising the manager of a hospital to detain someone when:

- the person has a mental disorder which causes their decision making to be 'significantly impaired';

- it is necessary as a matter of urgency to detain that person for assessment;
- either the person's health, safety or welfare, or the safety of another person, would be at significant risk if they were not detained;
- making arrangements for the possible granting of a short-term detention certificate would involve 'undesirable delay'.

Appendix 5.3	Key emergency detention orders (Source: Mental Health (Care and Treatment) Scotland Act 2003)		
MHA Order	**Purpose**	**Location**	**Duration**
Emergency detention	Urgent assessment by one fully registered doctor with (where possible consent of MHO where arranging short-term detention under order would cause unacceptable delay.	Hospital	Up to 72 hours
Short-term detention	Assessment or treatment by one AMP recommendation agreed by MHO.	Hospital	Up to 28 days*
Compulsory treatment	Urgent assessment from community following application by MHO, 2 AMP recommendations. Decision by Mental Health Trust.	Hospital or community	Up to 6 months*

*May be extended

GLOSSARY OF TERMS

Adrenergic Relating to adrenaline (epinephrine) or having a similar physiological effect to adrenaline

Advanced directive An advanced directive is a set of written instructions provided by the person in advance and states what treatments and help they want, or do not want.

Affect Observed external manifestation of emotion, how the individual appears to others

Affective disorder Mood disorder

Agnosia Loss of ability to recognise people, sound, objects, smells or other sensory stimuli not due to sensory loss

Akathisia A subjective feeling of restlessness resulting in an inability to sit or stay still or a need to pace

Anhedonia Inability to experience enjoyment in previously enjoyable activities

Antiadrenergic Antagonistic to the action of sympathetic or other adrenergic nerve fibres

Anticholinergic Blocks the effects of the neurotransmitter acetylcholine which is involved with learning and memory, glands and involuntary muscles

Antidopaminergic Prevents or counteracts the effects of dopamine

Antihistaminergic Counteracts the effects of histamine

Anxiety Subjective experience of worry or fear

Automatic negative thoughts Thoughts that come unbidden into consciousness and that affect mood or behaviour, e.g. 'they're not answering the door because they hate me'

Avoidance Avoiding situations or thoughts because they cause anxiety

Biopsychosocial model An approach suggesting that human functioning in disease or disorder is a combination of biological, psychological and social factors and suggests using a holistic/mind-body approach to treatment (Engel, 1977)

Blunted affect A limited range of emotional response where normal emotions are not present

Catatonia Extreme disorder of motor function, patients may sit still for hours or may show extreme motor activity and repetitive movements, bizarre posturing, echolalia, echopraxia and mutism. Occurs in catatonic schizophrenia

Cerebellar degeneration Relating to a process by which the neurons in the part of the brain that controls movement and balance - the cerebellum – degenerate or die causing impaired walking ability, tremors and balance problems

Cognitive behavioural therapy (CBT) CBT helps individuals to identify unhelpful and unrealistic thoughts and beliefs (cognitions) and behaviour patterns. Strategies to replace these with more positive and helpful thoughts and behaviours are identified and put into practice.

Community mental health team (CMHT) The CMHT is made up of a range of mental health professionals who deliver mental health services in the community. Key personnel are the psychiatrist, counsellor/psychologist, CPN, AMHP, OT and care coordinator.

Community psychiatric nurse (CPN) The role of the CPN is to support individuals with mental health conditions in the community. Individuals may have been discharged from a unit and part of the role of the CMHN is to support them and help avoid relapse or readmission into the psychiatric unit. They can also administer medication and injections.

Compulsions Repetitive, purposeful, physical or mental behaviours usually performed with reluctance in response to an obsession

Concentration Ability to maintain focus

Confabulation Falsified memory – patients may confabulate when they have no recollection of what actually happened

CRT Crisis resolution team

Cyclothymia Cycles of mania and depression over a two-year period that are less severe and do not meet the criteria for bipolar disorder

Disability Discrimination Act (DDA) Promotes civil rights for disabled people and protects disabled people from discrimination – www.Direct.gov.uk/Disability

'A person has a disability for the purposes of this Act if he has a physical or mental impairment which has a substantial and long-term adverse effect on his ability to carry out normal day-to-day activities.'
– www.opsi.gov.uk/acts/acts1995/ukpga_ 19950050_ en_2#pt1-l1g1

Delusion False, fixed or firmly held belief that is out of keeping with the culture/experience of the person and unchanged despite evidence to the contrary. Types include grandiose, persecutory, guilt, of reference, thought insertion, thought withdrawal, thought broadcast, passivity, somatic passivity, delusional perception and nihilistic.

Delusional perception A delusion that arises in response to a normal perception

Delusions of grandiosity The delusional belief that the person has special abilities, powers or is an important person

Delusions of guilt A delusional belief that the person has committed a crime or other terrible act. May occur in psychotic depression.

Delusions of jealousy/infidelity The delusional belief that a partner is unfaithful

Delusions of nihilism The delusional belief that the person has lost all their money or possessions or that they are dead and their body is rotting

Delusions of persecution The delusional belief that an organisation or person is trying to harm the person

Delusions of reference The delusional belief that events or situations have a particular meaning for the person, e.g. TV programmes are sending a message, cars parked there for a reason

Depersonalisation An unpleasant experience of subjective change, feeling detached, unreal, empty or emotionless, watching self from outside

Differential diagnosis A process where the likelihood of one condition is weighed against another condition to form a diagnosis, usually in cases where symptoms of different conditions may be similar

Dysfunctional (see also functional)
Deterioration (malfunction) of natural
processes that enable one to function
effectively e.g. a thought process, feeling or
behaviour

Disinhibition A loss of social conventions or
behaviour resulting in behaviour inappropriate
to the setting

Dissociative Psychological stress experienced as
physical (neurological) symptoms

Dopamine A neurotransmitter that affects the
way the brain controls movements and central
to the pleasure system of the brain. Shortage
causes Parkinson's disease. It is suggested that
dopamine pathways are altered in addiction

DSM Diagnostic and Statistical Manual of
Mental Disorders, the diagnostic tool for
mental health published by the American
Psychiatric Association

Dual diagnosis Meeting criteria for two
diagnoses simultaneously – usually a
psychiatric disorder and substance misuse
disorder

Dysthymia A period of low mood prevailing
over time but not severe enough to meet the
criteria for clinical depression

Echolalia Repeating words spoken by another
person, parrot fashion

Echopraxia Repeating actions of another person

**Eating disorders not otherwise specified
(EDNOS)** The diagnosis that may be given
to someone who is suffering from disordered
eating (e.g. calorie counting. Bingeing,
purging etc), but does not show all the
symptoms described by the 'text book'
definition of anorexia nervosa or bulimia
nervosa

Egodystonic A thought that is troublesome and
unwanted to the person who tries to resist it.
Obsessions are egodystonic

Electroconvulsive therapy (ECT) ECT
involves provoking seizures using a controlled
dose of electrical current in the brain

Euthymia Stable emotional state with normal
ups and downs

Extrapyramidal symptoms Movement side
effects of antipsychotic medications such as
Parkinsonism, bradykinesia, akathisia

First-rank symptoms (FRS) Originally devised
by Kurt Schnieder, these are important
diagnostic indicators of schizophrenia. FRS
include hallucinations, delusions, thought
insertion, removal and broadcasting

Flat affect An absence or near absence of an
appropriate emotional response in a situation
that would normally result in some form of
emotion

Flights of ideas Speech in which there is an
abnormal connection between statements –
based on rhyme or pun, not meaning

Formal thought disorder Speech indicates that
links between consecutive thoughts are not
meaningful, includes loosening of association

Frequency of Alcohol Scoring Test (FAST) A
four item test used to determine the presence
of hazardous or problem drinking

Functional (see also disfunctional) Processes
that enable an individual to conduct and
manage their regular activities, tasks and
relationships effectively e.g. a thought process,
feeling or behaviour

Grandiosity Patient's behaviour and speech
indicate a belief in superiority

Hallucination A perception in the absence of an external stimulus which is experienced as true and coming from the outside world

Health and Safety Executive (HSE) The national independent watchdog for work related health, safety and illness. They regulate and serve to act in the public interest to reduce work related injury, illness and deat across the UK

Ideas of reference Thoughts that others are looking at or talking about the person, not held with full delusional intensity

Illusion Distortion of a normal perception – seeing a rope as a snake

Incongruous affect Emotion expressed by the person is not what is expected in the situation – laughing at sad news

Interpersonal therapy (IPT) A problem-solving therapy that focuses on relationships with other people and on problems such as difficulties with communication or coping with bereavement

Loosening of associations Speech in which there is no discernable link between statements

Monoamine oxidase inhibitors (MAOIs) An older class of antidepressant used in cases where other medications have been ineffective. Can cause severe adverse reactions when taken with other medications or certain foods so are now less commonly used

Mood Subjective – a person's experience of their mental state

Objective Observed external manifestation of that state

The Mental Health Foundation (MHF) A charity that supports and campaigns for persons with mental health conditions – www.mentalhealth.org.uk

Morbid Thought or feeling held with such intensity and preoccupation that it causes significant distress

Negative symptoms Symptoms characterised by loss of normal function

Neologism Made-up words (e.g. foothat for shoe), a second rank symptom of schizophrenia

Neuroleptic malignant syndrome Potentially fatal complication of antipsychotics causing hyperpyrexia (increased set body temperature), autonomic instability, confusion and increased muscle tone

Neurosis Mental distress where the ability to distinguish between the person's mind and external reality is retained. Covers most depressive/anxiety disorders

The National Insitute for Health and Clinical Excellence (NICE) is an independent organisation responsible for providing national clinical guidance (published and in development) on promoting good health and preventing and treating ill health – www.nice.org.uk

The National Institute of Mental Health (NIMH) An organisation in the USA whose mission is to transform the understanding and treatment of mental illnesses through basic and clinical research, paving the way for prevention, recovery, and cure

Obsession Recurrent thoughts, feelings, impulses or images that are intrusive, senseless, persistent and unwelcome, but recognised as their own

Othello Syndrome The overwhelming delusion of a partner/spouse's infidelity. Often seen in substance abuse and schizophrenia

Outcome expectancy The expected positive and negative outcome of action or inaction

Panic attack Period of fear, impending doom or discomfort accompanied by somatic symptoms

Passivity Being passive, submissive, inactive or acquiescent

Perceptive selectivity Processing only some of the stimuli or information being experienced. For example, if we are hungry we see food shops not shoe shops

Phobia Fear or anxiety out of proportion to the situation, leading to avoidance

Positive symptoms Symptoms of schizophrenia characterised by abnormal thoughts and perceptions such as hallucinations and delusions

Pressure of speech Rate and volume of speech are increased so it is difficult to interrupt

Psychomotor agitation Increase in overall motor activity occurring in mania

Psychomotor retardation Decrease in overall motor activity occurring in depression

Psychosis Severe mental disturbance characterised by a loss of contact with external reality. Delusions, hallucinations and disorganised thinking are often present

Reversible inhibitors of monoamine oxidase (RIMAs) A selective type of antidepressant from the drug group MAOI

The Scottish Association for Mental Health (SAMH) The leading mental health charity in Scotland

Second-rank symptoms (SRS) SRS occur in both schizophrenia and other mental health disorders such as mania and include some types of delusions and hallucinations

Selective serotonin reuptake inhibitors (SSRIs) A group of antidepressants which maintain circulating levels of serotonin to help alleviate depressive symptoms

Self-efficacy An individual's perceived confidence regarding their ability to perform a specific action, behaviour or task

Serotonin Also called 5-hydroxytryptamine (5-HTP), found in the pineal gland, blood platelets, the digestive tract, and brain. It acts as a messenger that transmits nerve signals between nerve cells. Changes in brain levels can alter the mood

Somatic passivity The delusion that an outside force is able to control bodily functions

Somatoform disorders A mental health condition characterised by physical symptoms arising from psychological factors, for example hypochondriasis or body dysmorphic disorder

Splitting A defence mechanism that involves separating in the mind the positive and negative qualities of self/others, people are perceived as all good or all bad

Stereotypy Repetitive, purposeless movements (e.g. rocking)

Tardive dyskinesia A side effect (often permanent) of typical antipsychotics that involves repetitive purposeless movements, often of the face

Tricyclic antidepressants (TCAs) An older antidepressant group, now less frequently used due to severity of side effects

Thought block A subjective experience that thoughts suddenly disappear

Thought broadcasting The delusional belief that thoughts are available to others, may include the belief that thoughts are being broadcast to others or are known by telepathy

Thought echo An auditory hallucination where the person hears their thoughts spoken out loud

Thought insertion Experiencing thoughts as alien and not one's own with the belief that they have been inserted by an external force

Thought withdrawal The delusional belief that thoughts are being removed by an external force

REFERENCES

Abi-Dargham, A. et al. (2000) 'Increased baseline occupancy of D 2 receptors by dopamine in schizophrenia', *Proceedings of the National Academy of Sciences* (PNAS), 97:8104–9

ACSM (2010) ACSM's *Guidelines for Exercise Testing and Prescription*, 8th edn., USA, Lippincott, Williams and Wilkins

Addiction alternatives (2010) 'Relapse prevention strategies'. Accessed from: www.addictionalternatives. com/philosophy/relapseprevention.htm Accessed: 6 September 2010

Agras, W.S.,Walsh, B.T., Fairburn, C.G. et al. (2000) 'A multicentre comparison of cognitive-behavioural therapy and interpersonal psychotherapy for bulimia nervosa', *Archives of General Psychiatry*, 57:459–66

Almond, P. (2009) 'Postnatal depression: A global public health perspective', *Perspectives in Public Health*, 5:221–7. Accessed from: www.sagepub.com Accessed: October 2009

American Psychological Association (APA) (2000) *The Diagnostic and Statistical Manual of Mental Disorders*, USA, American Psychiatric Association

British Association for Cancer Research (BACR) (1997) *Exercise Instructor Training Manual – Cardiac Rehabilitation Module*, UK, Human Kinetics Europe Ltd

Baker-Brown, S. (2006) 'A patient's journey: Living with paranoid schizophrenia', *BMJ*, 333:636–8, doi: 10.1136/bmj.38968.608275.AE

Bacaltchuk, J., Hay, P., Trefiglio, R. (2001) 'Antidepressants versus psychological treatments and their combination for bulimia nervosa', *Cochrane Database of Systematic Reviews. Accessed from http://www.ncbi.nlm.nih.gov/pubmed Accessed on 19 December 2010*

Bayne, R et al. (1998) *The Counsellor's Handbook*, UK, Nelson Thomas

Bean, A. (2010) *Sports Nutrition for Women*, UK, A & C Black Ltd

Bentau, R. (2010) Doctoring the Mind: Why psychiatric treatments fail, UK, Penguin Books

Bess, M. PhD, Albrecht, A. RN, MS, King, T. PhD, Parisi, A. MD, Pinto, B. PhD, Roberts, M. MS, Niaura R. PhD, Abrams, B. PhD (1999) 'The efficacy of exercise as an aid for smoking cessation in women a randomized controlled trial', *Archives of Internal Medicine*, 159:1229–34

Bird, W. (2007) Natural Thinking: A Report by Dr William Bird, for the Royal Society for the Protection of Birds investigating the links between the natural environment, biodiversity and mental health. Accessed from: www.rspb.org.uk/policy/health Accessed on: 18 November 2010

Borg, G. (1998) *Perceived Exertion and Pain Scales*, USA, Human Kinetics

Boyes, C. (2005) *Need to Know? Body Language*, UK, Collins

British National Formulary (2005) 'Joint National Formulary Committee. British National Formulary' *London: British Medical Association and Royal Pharmaceutical Society of Great Britain*, 50th edn. Accessed from: www.bnf.org.uk Accessed on: 22 September 2005

British Nutrition Foundation (2005) 'Balance of Good Health' Accessed from: www.nutrition.org.uk Accessed on 24 November 2005

Benson, H. MD (1975) *The Relaxation Response*. USA, Avon Books

Biddle, S.J.H., Fox, K. & Boutcher, S., eds (2000) *Physical Activity and Psychological Well-being*, UK and USA, Routledge

Biddle, S.J.H., Mutrie, N. (revised 2008) *Psychology of Physical Activity*, USA, Routledge,

Boud, D., Keogh, R. & Walker, D. eds (1985) *Reflection: Turning experience into Learning*, London, UK, Kogan Page

British Heart Foundation (BHF) (2009) *Physical Activity and Health Factsheet*, UK, BHF

British Crime Survey (2006/7) Accessed from: http://rds.homeoffice.gov.uk/rds/bcs1.html Accessed on 11 November 2010

Blyn, L. et al. (1992) 'Schizophrenia and city life', *The Lancet*, 340(8812):137

Breier, A. et al. (1997) 'Schizophrenia is associated with elevated amphetamine-induced synaptic dopamine concentrations: Evidence from a novel positron emission tomography method', *PNAS* 94:2569–74

Buka, S.L. et al. (2001) 'Maternal infections and subsequent psychosis among offspring', *Archives of General Psychiatry*, 58(11):1032–7

Canadian Society for Exercise Physiology (2002) 'Screening forms: Physical activity readiness questionnaire and physical activity readiness medical examination', Accessed from: www.csep.ca/ Accessed on: 18 October 2005

Cantopher, T (2003) *Depressive illness: The curse of the strong*. UK, Sheldon Press

Carr, A. (2001) *Abnormal Psychology*, UK, Psychology Press

Chopra, A.K., Doody, G.A. (2007) 'Crime rates and local newspaper coverage of schizophrenia', *The Psychiatrist*, 31:206–8

Costin, C. (1997) *The Eating Disorder Source Book*, USA, RGA Publishing Group

Cox, J.L. et al. (1993) 'A controlled study of the onset, duration and prevalence of postnatal depression', *The British Journal of Pyschiatry*, 163:27–31

Crone, D., Heaney, L., Herbert, R., Morgan, J., Johnston, L., Macpherson, R. (2004) 'A comparison of lifestyle behaviour and health perceptions of people with severe mental illness and the general population', *Journal of Public Mental Health*, 3(4):19–25

Crown copyright (2010) *Mental Health First Aid Manual, Wales*, Mind Cymru and Welsh Assembly Government

Daines, B., Gask, L. & Usherwood, T. (1997) *Medical and Psychiatric Issues for Counsellors*, UK, Sage Publications

Davies, T. & Craig, T., eds (2009) *ABC of Mental Health*, UK, Wiley Blackwell

Davison, G. & Neale, J. (2001) *Abnormal Psychology*, 8th edn., USA, John Wiley & Sons

Deci, E.L. & Ryan, R.M. (1985) *Intrinsic Motivation and Self-determination in Human Behavior*, USA, Plenum

Deci, E.L. & Ryan, R.M. (2000) 'The "what" and "why" of goal pursuits: Human needs and the self-determination of behavior', *Psychological Inquiry*, 11:227–68

Delisle, T.T., Werch, C.E., Wong, A.H., Bian, H., Weiler, R.(March 2010) 'Relationship between frequency and intensity of physical activity and health behaviors of adolescents', *Journal of School Health*, 80(3):134–40

Department of Health (DoH) (1999) 'National Service Framework', UK, DoH Accessed from: www.dh.gov.uk Accessed on: 16 June 2011

DoH (2001). *Exercise Referral Systems: A National Quality Assurance Framework*, UK, DoH

DoH (2004) *At Least Five a Week: Evidence on the impact of physical activity and its relationship to health. A report from the Chief Medical Officer*, UK, DoH

DoH (2004b) *Choosing Health: Making healthier choices easier*, UK, DoH

DoH (2005) *Choosing Activity: A physical activity action plan*, UK, DoH

DoH (2011) '*No health without mental health: A cross government mental health outcomes strategy for people of all ages*', 9. Accessed from: http://www.dh.gov.uk/en/Healthcare/MentalHealth/MentalHealthStrategy/index.htm Accessed on: 16 February 2011

DeVries, H.A. (1981) 'Tranquiliser effects of exercise; a critical review', *Physician and Sports Medicine*, 9:46–55

Durstine, L.J. & Moore, G. (2003) *ACSM's Exercise Management for Persons with Chronic Diseases and Disabilities*, 2nd edn., USA, Human Kinetics

Eating Disorders online (2011) Eating disorders not otherwise specified. Accessed from: http://www.eatingdisordersonline.com/explain/ednos.php Accessed on: 22 February 2011

Ellin, J. (1994) *Listening Helpfully: How to develop your counselling skills*, UK, Souvenir Press.

Eisler, I., Dare, C., Russell, G.F.M. et al. (1997) 'Family and individual therapy in anorexia nervosa', *Archives of General Psychiatry*, 54:1025–30

Eisler, I., Dare, C., Hodes, M. et al. (2000) 'Family therapy for anorexia nervosa in adolescents: the results of a controlled comparison of two family interventions', *Journal of Child Psychology and Psychiatry*, 41:727–36

Eleverton, P (2004) *Taming the Black Dog*, Oxford, UK, How To books

Engel, G. L. (1977) 'The need for a new medical model: A challenge for biomedicine'. *Science* 196:129–136

Fairburn, C.G., Norman, P.A., Welch, S.L. et al. (1995) 'A prospective study of outcome in bulimia nervosa and the long-term effects of three psychological treatments', *Archives of General Psychiatry*, 52:304–12

Faulkner, G. & Taylor, A., eds (2005) *Exercise, Health and Mental Health: Emerging relationships*, UK, Routledge

Feltham, C. & Horton, I., eds (2000) *Handbook of Counselling and Psychotherapy*, UK, Sage Publications

Fernando, S. (1988) *Race and Culture in Psychiatry*, UK, Croom Helm

Fox, K., ed. (1997) *The Physical Self*, USA, Human Kinetics

Fox, K. (1997) 'Mirror, mirror'. Accessed from: www.sirc.org/publik/mirror.html Accessed on: 21 December 2010

General Practice Notebook, 'A UK medical encyclopaedia on the web', Accessed from: www.gpnotebook.co.uk Accessed on: 2 October 2005

Grant, T. (2000) *Physical Activity and Mental Health*, UK, Health Education Authority

Gross, R. & McIlveen, R. (1998) *Psychology: A new introduction*, London, Hodder and Stoughton

Hay, P.J. & Bacaltchuk, J. (2001) 'Psychotherapy for bulimia nervosa and bingeing', Cochrane Review in *The Cochrane Library*, (1)

Halliwell, E. (2005) 'Up and Running? Exercise therapy and the treatment of mild or moderate depression in primary care', UK. Accessed from: www.mentalhealth. org.uk Accessed on: 18 July 2005

Hamer, M. Stamatakis, E., Steptoe, A. (2008) 'Dose-response relationship between physical activity and mental health: the Scottish Health Survey.' *British Journal of Sports Medicine* 10 April 2008

Hays, K., (1999) *Working it out: Using exercise in psychotherapy*, VA, USA American Psychiatric Association

Hawkins, N. (November 2009) 'Battling our bodies: Understanding and overcoming negative body images'. Accessed from: ezinearticles.com/?expert=Nicole_Hawkins,_Ph.D. Accessed on: 21 December 2010

Health Development Agency (HDA) (2005) 'Getting evidence into practice in public health'. Accessed from: www.had.nhs.uk Accessed on: 25 August 2005

HDA (2005) 'Choosing health? Choosing activity: Comments on the consultation document from the health development agency'. Accessed from: www.had. nhs.uk Accessed on: 25 August 2005

Hendrix, M. (1994) 'Anxiety disorders'. Accessed from: www.nimh.nih.gov/publicat/anxiety.cfm Accessed on: 18 July 2005

Health and Safety Executive (HSE) (2002/3) 'Occupational Health Statistics Bulletin UK'. Accessed from: www. hse.gov.uk/statistics/pdf/swi8p5.pdf Accessed on: 23 July 2005

HSE (2003) 'Five Steps to Risk Assessment'. Available from: www.hse.gov.uk. Accessed on: 10 December 2005

HSE (2005) 'Stress related and psychological disorders'. Accessed from: www.hse.gov.uk/statistics/causdis/ stress.htm Accessed on: 23 July 2005

Health Education Authority (HEA) (1997) *Mental Health Promotion: A quality framework*, UK, HEA

HEA (2005) 'Executive summary', UK. Accessed from: www.had-online.org.uk Accessed in: October 2005

HEA (2000) 'Black and minority ethnic groups in England: The second health and lifestyles survey' in 'Executive summary', UK. Accessed from: www.had-online.org.uk Accessed on: 20 October 2005

Health Survey for England (2008) Department of Health, UK

Hughes, J. & Martin, S. (1999) in (Waine, C. 2002) *Obesity and Weight Management in Primary Care*, UK, Blackwell Publishing

Idzikowski, C. (date) The Insomnia Kit: Practical Advice for a Good Night's Sleep

International Physical Activity Questionnaire (2002) Available from: www.ipaq.ki.se Accessed on: 18 November 2005

Jackson, C. & Hill, K., eds, (2006) *Mental Health Today: A handbook*, UK, Pavilion Publishing in conjunction with the Mental Health Foundation. (MHF)

Joint Health Surveys Unit (2003) *Health Survey for England*, UK, The Stationary Office

Joint Health Surveys Unit (1999) *Health Survey for England: Health of minority ethnic groups*, UK, The Stationary Office

Jonas, S. & Phillips, E. (2009) *ACSM's Exercise is Medicine: A clinicians guide to exercise prescription*, USA, Lippincott, Williams and Wilkins

Johnston D. & Mayers, C. (2005) 'Spirituality: A review of how occupational therapists acknowledge, assess and meet spiritual needs', British Journal of Occupational Therapy, 68(9): 386

Lago, C. & Thompson, J. (2003) *Race, Culture and Counselling*, UK, Open University Press

Lawrence, D. (2004) *The Complete Guide to Exercise to Music*, 2nd edn., UK, A & C Black Publishers Ltd.

Lawrence, D. (2004) *The Complete Guide to Exercise in Water*, 2nd edn., UK, A & C Black Publishers Ltd.

Lawrence, D. & Bolitho S. (2011) *Exercise Your Way to Health: Stress*, UK, A & C Black Publishers Ltd.

Lawrence, D. & Hope, B. (2005) *The Complete Guide to Circuit Training*, UK, A & C Black Publishers Ltd.

Lawrence, D. (2005) *The Complete Guide to Exercising Away Stress*, UK, A & C Black Publishers Ltd.

Lawrence, D. & Barnett, L. (2006) *GP Referral Schemes*, UK, A & C Black Publishers Ltd.

Leith, L.M. (1994) *Foundations of Exercise and Mental Health*, USA, Fitness Information Technology

Linde K., Berner, M.M., Kriston, L. (2008) 'St John's wort for major depression', *Cochrane Database of Systematic Reviews*, (4)

Lowe, B., Zipfel, S., Buchholz, C., Dupont, Y., Reas, D.L. & Herzog, W. (2001) 'Long-term outcome of anorexia nervosa in a prospective 21-year follow-up study', *Psychological Medicine*, 31:881–90

Luck, A.J., Morgan, J.F., Reid, F. et al. (2002) 'The SCOFF questionnaire and clinical interview for eating disorders in general practice: Comparative study', *British Medical Journal*, 325:755–6

Martinsen, E.W. (1993) 'Therapeutic implications of exercise for clinically anxious and depressed clients', *International Journal of Sport Psychology*, 24:185–99

McArdle, W., Katch, F. & Katch, V. (1991) *Exercise Physiology: Energy, nutrition and human performance*, USA, Lea and Febiger

Menezes, P.R. et al. (1996) 'Drug and alcohol problems among individuals with severe mental illness in south London', *British Journal of Psychiatry*, 168:612–9

Mental Health Foundation (MHF) (2007) *Fundamental Facts*, UK, Mental Health Foundation

MHF (2010) *Mindfulness Report*, UK, Mental Health Foundation

MHF (2010) 'Mental health problems', UK, MHF. Accessed from: www.mentalhealth.org.uk/information/mental-health-overview/mental-health-problems/?locale=en Accessed on: 6 September 2010

Millett, K. (1991) *The Loony Bin Trip*, UK, Virago Press

Milos, G., Spindler A., Schnyder, U. & Fairburn, C.G. 'Instability of eating disorder diagnoses: prospective study', *British Journal of Psychiatry*, 187:573–8

Mindell, A. (1995) *Sitting in the Fire: Large group transformation using conflict and diversity*, USA, Lao Tse Press

Moore, T.H.M. et al. (2007) 'Cannabis use and risk of psychotic or affective mental health outcomes: A systematic review', *The Lancet*, 370(9584):319–28

Mueser, K.T. & McGurk, S.R. (2004) Schizophrenia, *The Lancet*, 363(9426):2063–72

Mulvany, F. et al. (2001) 'Effect of social class at birth on risk and presentation of schizophrenia: Case-control study', *British Medical Journal*, 323:1398–401, doi: 10.1136/bmj.323.7326.1398

Morgan, W. P. & Goldston, S.E. (1987) *Exercise and Mental Health*, USA, Hemisphere

NHS (2001) Exercise Referral Systems: A National Quality Assurance Framework (NAQF), Department of Health, UK

National Treatment Agency (2009) www.nta.nhs.uk/areas/facts_and_figures/0708/default.aspx. Office for National Statistics. Accessed from: www.statistics.gov.uk/cci/nugget.asp?id=313 Accessed on: 21 February 2011

Neal, M.J. (2002) *Medical Pharmacology at a Glance*, UK, Blackwell Publishing

National Institute for Health and Clinical Excellence (NICE) (2006) *Schizophrenia: Full national clinical guideline on core interventions in primary and secondary care*, UK, NICE

NICE (2009) *Depression: Guidelines 90–91: Quick reference guide*, UK, NICE

NICE (2009) *Anxiety: Management of anxiety in adults in primary, secondary and community care: Clinical guideline 22 amended*, UK, NICE

National Institute of Mental Health (NIMH) (2010) 'Schizophrenia'. Accessed from: www.nimh.nih.gov/health/publications/schizophrenia/complete-index.shtml Accessed on: 7 September 2010

Office for National Statistics (2007) 'Alcohol-related deaths by occupation, England and Wales, 2001– 05', *Health Statistics Quarterly*, 35, ONS, UK

Owen, M.J., O'Donovan, M.C. & Harrison, P.J. (2005) 'Schizophrenia: A genetic disorder of the synapse?' *British Medical Journal*, 330:158–9, doi: 10.1136/bmj.330.7484.158

Peen, J. & Dekker, J. (2004) 'Is urbanicity an environmental risk-factor for psychiatric disorders?' *The Lancet*, 363(9426):2012–3

Petty, G. (2004) *Teaching Today*, 3rd edn, UK, Nelson Thornes

Phelps, S. & Austin, N. (1997) *The Assertive Women*, 3rd edn, Impact Publishers Inc, US

Plante, T.G. (1996) 'Getting physical: Does exercise help in the treatment of psychiatric disorders?' *Journal of Psychosocial Nursing*, 43(3):38–43

PRODIGY (2005) 'Depression'. Available from: www.prodigy.nhs.uk Accessed on: 28 August 2005

Rack, P. (1982) *Race, Culture and Mental Disorder*, UK, Tavistock

Rassool, G.H. (2009) *Alcohol and Drug Misuse*, UK, Routledge

Rethink (2006) 'Schizophrenia', UK, National Advice Service factsheet

Rethink (2010) 'Scizoaffective disorder', UK, National Advice Service factsheet. Accessed from: http://www.rethink.org/about_mental_illness/mental_illnesses_and_disorders/schizoaffective_disorder/index.html Accessed on: 23 February 2011

Rogers, C. & Stevens, B. (1967) *Person to Person: The problem of being human*, USA, Real People Press

Royal College of Psychiatrists (2009) The Young Mind: An essential guide to mental health for young adults, parents and teachers, UK, Bantam Press

Royal College of Psychiatrists (2004) Schizophrenia, UK, Bantam Press

Royal Society of Psychiatrists (2011) 'Eating disorders'. Accessed from: http://www.rcpsych.ac.uk/mentalhealthinfoforall/problems/eatingdisorders/eatingdisorders.aspx. Accessed on: 23 February 2011

Royal College of Psychiatrists (2009) *Eating Well Leaflet.* RCP, UK

Royal College of Psychiatrists (2010) Post Natal Depression. Accessed from www.rcpsych.ac.uk/mentalhealth infoforall/problems/postnatalmentalhealth/ postnataldepression. Accessed on: 19 December 2010

Ryan, R.M., & Deci, E.L. (2000) 'Self-determination theory and the facilitation of intrinsic motivation, social development, and well-being', *American Psychologist*, 55:68–78

Sainsbury Centre for Mental Health (2003) 'Economic and social costs of mental illness in England', UK. Accessed from: www.scmh.org.uk Accessed on: 19 December 2010

Scott, J., (2001) 'Cognitive behavioural therapy as adjunct to medication in bipolar disorder', *British Journal of Psychiatry*, 178:164–8

Semple, D., Smyth, R., Burns, J., Darjee, R., McIntosh, A. (2005) *Oxford Handbook of Psychiatry*, UK, Oxford University Press

Senior, R., Barnes, J., Emberson, J.R. & Golding, J. on behalf of the ALSPAC Study Team (2005) 'Early experiences and their relationship to maternal eating disorder symptoms, both lifetime and during pregnancy', *British Journal of Psychiatry*, 187:268–73

Sinyor, D. et al. (1982) 'The role of a physical fitness program in the treatment of alcoholism', *Journal of Studies on Alcohol*, 43(3):380–6

Smith, C.A, Hay, P.P.J., MacPherson, H. (2010) 'Acupuncture for depression', *Cochrane Database of Systematic Reviews* 1: CD004046. DOI: 10.1002/14651858.CD004046.pub3.

Spearing, M. (1999) Depression. Accessed from: http://www.nimh.nih.gov/publicat/depression.cfm. Accessed on: 21 February 2011

Spearing, M. (2001) 'Eating disorders: Facts about eating disorders and the search for solutions', USA. Accessed from: www.nimh.nih.gov/publicat/eatingdisorders.cfm Accessed on: 18 July 2005

Spearing, M. (2002) 'Bipolar disorder', USA. Accessed from: www.nimh.nih.gov/publicat/bipolar.cfm Accessed on: 18 July 2005

Spearing, M. (2009) 'Schozophrenia'. Accessed from: http://www.nimh.nih.gov/health/publications/ schizophrenia/complete-index.shtml Accessed on: 22 February 2011

Stefan, M., Travis, M. & Murray, R.M., eds, (2002) An *Atlas of Schizophrenia*, UK, Parthenon Publishing

Stewart, I. & Joines, V. (1987) *TA Today: A new introduction to transactional analysis*, UK, Lifespace Publishing

Strock, M. (2000) 'Depression', USA. Accessed from: www.nimh.nih.gov/publicat/depression.cfm Accessed on: 18 July 2005

Evans, R. (2009) *Qualitative Evaluation of Sustrans 'Bike it– Walk it' Initiative in the South Wales Valleys*, UK, Sustrans/Integrate Consulting

Theander, S. (1985) 'Outcome and prognosis in anorexia nervosa and bulimia: Some results of previous investigations compared with those of a Swedish long-term study', *Journal of Psychiatric Research*, 19:493–508

Turner, T. (1997) 'ABC of mental health: Schizophrenia', *British Medical Journal*, 315:108–11

Tetrault, J. MD, Crothers, K. MD, Moore, B. PhD, Mehra, R. MD, Concato, J. MD, MS, MPH, Fiellin, D. MD (2007) 'Effects of marijuana smoking on pulmonary function and respiratory complications: A systematic review', Archives of Internal Medicine, 167(3):221–8

The Health and Social Care Information Centre (2008) *Lifestyles Statistics*, NHS, UK

University of Rochester (Date unknown) 'Self-determination theory'. Accessed from: www.psych.rochester.edu/SDT/ theory.php Accessed on: 16 August 2010

U.S. Department of Health and Human Sciences (2008) *Physical Activity Guidelines for Americans*, USA, HSS

Van de Weyer, C. (2005) 'Changing diets, changing minds: How food affects mental well-being and behaviour', Accessed from: www.mentalhealthfoundation.co.uk Accessed on: 16 November 2010

Waine, C. (2002) *Obesity and Weight Management in Primary Care*, UK, Blackwell Publishing

Web MD Corporation (2001) Understanding Schizophrenia, Accessed from: www.wfmh.org/PDF/ schizophrenia Accessed on: 23 February 2010

Websters New World Dictionary (1986) *The New International Websters Comprehensive Dictionary of the English Language. Encyclopedic Edition*. Florida, USA, Trident Press

Winnail, S.D., Valois, R.F., McKeown, R.E, Saunders R.P, Pate, R.R (1995) 'Relationship between physical activity level and cigarette, smokeless tobacco, and marijuana use among public high school adolescents', *Journal of School Health*, 65(10): 438–42

World Health Organisation (WHO) (1993) *The ICD-10 International Classification of Mental and Behavioural Disorders*, WHO

INDEX